WEIGHT LOS

JANET THOMSON MSc

WEIGHT LOSS
IN
MIND

Matador
5 Weir Road
Kibworth Beauchamp
Leicester LE8 0LQ, UK
Tel: (+44) 116 279 2299
Email: books@troubador.co.uk
Web: www.troubador.co.uk/matador

ISBN 978 1906510 350

Typeset in 11pt Skia by Troubador Publishing Ltd, Leicester, UK
Printed in the UK by TJ International, Padstow, Cornwall

Matador is an imprint of Troubador Publishing Ltd

CONTENTS

ACKNOWLEDGEMENTS

I am so blessed to have so many people in my life who have inspired me and that have helped me (some are not even aware of how much!) in my quest to bring you the best ever weight loss book. I will include some of them here, but the rest ... you know who you are.

Thank you to Sean Quigley. You are my soulmate.

Huge thanks to Igor at Venture Portraits Leicester for the wonderful cover shots (front and back) and the TFT pictures inside. Thank you also to the talented Luke Martin for his excellent cartoons. Thanks also to Joy and Gez Martin for being my health and fitness "Guru's" and great friends.

Thank you to Lyn Churcher and Sarah Braund at Churcher Associates, for always believing in me. Thanks and appreciation to Stephen and Louise Fordham at Essensuals (Rugby), for the great hair cuts, the ongoing support, and of course for making me laugh. After all it's Ok to feel good for no reason whatsoever... right?

To Deirdre Randall and Ramona Baretto... the best friends a girl can have.

My mum and dad, Ken and Rita Eagle, have always believed that everything I write deserves a Nobel Prize!

My fantastic children Ben Ryan and Emilie have taught me more about life than everyone else put together. Thank you seems inadequate.

IMPORTANT NOTE

In NLP conversation (written or spoken) the sentences are often formed or punctuated differently than in "traditional" English Grammar: This is to enable the brain to process the information in a more productive way. Therefore any grammatical errors you may or not notice may or may not be intentional.

ARE YOU READY TO CHANGE?

You want to lose weight or you wouldn't be reading this book: You are not happy with how you look, feel or both and you want to be different from how you are now. You want to change – but you don't know how. Chances are you have tried other "diets" and either failed miserably or succeeded short term only to put the weight straight back on plus a few more pounds for good measure. Depressing wasn't it?

What I would like you to do for the time being is suspend all "beliefs" you have about what works and what doesn't and be open to try something completely different, something new that is based on changing how you THINK rather than just what you eat. After all if you didn't "think" you wanted a bar of chocolate or an extra slice of pizza, you wouldn't eat it!

This is not a book you just read, it is a book you DO, you are not going to be a passive reader you will be an active participant. Think of it like a children's activity book without the colouring in! I can and will show you the exercises to do, but YOU HAVE TO DO THEM! You can achieve whatever you want to....... yes even that. Excited? YES you will be.

Crazy as it sounds if you pretend it works even before you start it works, even better. There is no programme that works for everyone, but the success rate for this plan is extremely high: in fact it works for EVERYONE who does actually DO IT, as opposed to just read it. If you are a bit nervous about trying something new – good! That will make you be more inquisitive. When you were a child you were naturally curious, that's how you learnt so much in such a short space of time. Approach this programme like a child learning a new skill: children like to try and experience everything, to prove to themselves things really happen. Tell a child not to touch something as it's hot and most of them reach out and touch it, just to prove it to themselves, at least until they learn better! So go back to your childhood way of learning, which is to have as much fun as possible and gain information that will help you now and in the future. A weight loss book that is fun? Now there's a first!!

If you feel confused at times that's FANTASTIC: confusion means your brain is working and accepting new information that it hasn't had before and trying to put it into some kind of filing system or programme where it can be accessed. Richard Bandler the co creator of NLP (Neuro Linguistic Programming) describes confusion as *"An opportunity to rearrange experience and organise it in a different way than you normally would. That allows you to learn to do something new and see and hear the world in a new way"*. Confusion comes before understanding.

You may find that when you are not reading this, your mind is busy filing away what you have learnt in an order that works for you. You will probably find yourself thinking about stuff you have read for no apparent reason, perhaps when you are at work or in the middle of the supermarket. Maybe you will begin to daydream as you process new ways of thinking.

Where shall we start? There's so much to learn about how your brain works and how you are driven towards making certain choices and developing certain behaviours, it is going to be exciting finding out what makes *you* tick.

Although we are all different (thank goodness!) there are some traits that we all have in common and one of those is our basic decision making process. Many psychologists talk about the "Pleasure or Pain" concept which helps you recognise patterns in your behaviour. Let me explain:

PLEASURE OR PAIN?

When you get up in the morning, what motivates you to get out of bed? Do you lie there for as long as you can until the unpleasant consequences of not getting up e.g. being late for work, or being late getting the children to school, become a real possibility, or do you leap out of bed thinking the sooner you get up the more time you will have to get ready, or that you will have time for that cooked breakfast.

Both of these are based on different motivation strategies that influence everything you do: every decision you make is influenced by whether it will cause you pleasure or pain. Imagine a sliding scale with one end being PAIN and the other PLEASURE.

Pain - quite bad - OK quite good - good

MASSIVE PAIN 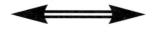 **INTENSE PLEASURE**

The distance in between is varying scales or levels of these feelings, for example just over the $\frac{1}{2}$ way line towards "pleasure" is feeling "quite good", then it moves towards feeling very good, then "really great" and so on up until "INTENSE PLEASURE" reaches its peak at the right end of the line. In the same way moving in the other direction you may have "feeling slightly down, fed up, depressed" and so on until "MASSIVE PAIN" is left at the other end of the line.

If you associate massive PAIN with something, you are unlikely to do it, in fact you will take action to avoid doing it. On the other hand if you think it will bring you pleasure you are likely to do it willingly and with positive expectations.

We can apply this principle to all decisions, even though we may be unaware of it. This story of a client who came to me for coaching a couple of years ago:

Jane had been working in an office for a couple of years and the job was OK. She was working with a group of people most of whom she got on with, but her boss could be really stroppy at times and when he asked her to do something he rarely said please or thank you. It's a little thing that she noticed and at first it didn't bother her, but after a while it began to grate and she started to feel really unappreciated. Her first steps towards Pain. One day he once again told her to do something just as she was finishing work, she did it but felt resentful as he had encroached into her personal time and he didn't even say please or thank you. She thought about it all the way home, getting more and more annoyed and eventually decided enough was enough and that she had to look for another job: she was moving further towards pain on the scale. That night she got the local paper and went through the internet looking for suitable jobs in her area. She was surprised to find there was not much out there that would suit her, but she did find some positions that might be OK. She typed an up to date C.V. and sent it off. She went to work feeling better as she new she wasn't going to stay in that situation for much longer. Just knowing she was doing something about it made her feel better. However, after a week or so when the rejection letters started to come through, she began to feel disappointed and that knocked her confidence somewhat, causing pain. A week later she got a call from a company that wanted her to attend an interview, she moved back towards pleasure as the prospect of a new start loomed: the day arrived and she spent ages deciding what to wear as everything she had she thought made her look fat/frumpy etc.(more Pain). She went to the interview and really undersold herself due to lack of confidence and didn't get the job even though she knew she was the ideal candidate. Jane then experienced rejection, low self esteem and **Massive Pain.** The thought of another interview and more rejection compounded this feeling. She couldn't face it.

She went into work the next day and thought "Well its not so bad here, most of the people are nice and so what if the boss never says please, its not my fault he is a miserable git, the rest of the staff are nice, I'll stay here". So she settled back into her less painful life. She settled for less than she wanted because the process of change was too painful, you could say the cure became worse than the disease, she gave up. She moved away from Pain and towards the safety of what she knew. Even though it was not the "Pleasure" she was after it was not as bad as the pain of being in the job market. She settled for less.

Have you ever settled for less? Do you settle for less? Are you prepared to settle for less?

Let's put it into context for where you are at now: have you ever "dieted" before? If not do you know anyone who has repeatedly tried to lose weight and failed? If this is the case, as it is for most everyone, then you may have very strong negative associations with dieting that represent massive pain. At the moment you are unhappy with how you look, you are in your opinion too fat. *(I prefer not to use the term overweight even though its more politically correct, I know you don't look in the mirror and say "I look a little bit overweight today" you look in the mirror and you say "I am fat" so its important we talk the same language).* Feeling like this causes you pain and reduces your confidence and self esteem. You will do what you can to avoid pain so you decide to do something about it. You pick up the paper/magazine and start the latest quick fix diet. You start off really positive, this one *will* work. After a week or so you realise you don't like many of the foods, after all separating and eating pure egg white and having it on on toast without butter isn't the most appealing meal. It also means cooking different meals for yourself than others in the house (or risk them all moaning), perhaps you feel hungry much of the time and miss the foods you are "not allowed". Within a short space of time the diet becomes so *painful* that you realise you were much happier before you started, so you go back to your previous eating and lifestyle which is less painful. You give up on the concept of achieving the Pleasure you associate with being lighter because the "cure" in this case "diet" is worse (more painful) than being fat. You have settled for less than you really want.

Even before you started this book, the very fact that you bought it shows that you are in "pain" with your shape or size at the moment. This is good as it has motivated you to take action now, so what you need from here on is a programme that doesn't involve pain. A way of making changes that you actually enjoy. Read on.

You can learn how to reprogram your mind to only eat when

you are hungry and to find the foods that made you fat repulsive, how does that make you feel? Can you see yourself achieving your goals? Think about it for a moment, really visualise how that would look and feel. To only eat foods you enjoy and only eat as much as you need, not as much as you used to want. Imagine you have already been doing this for a few weeks and are really loving your food and you can already see a difference in your shape, your clothes are looser your flabby bits getting firmer – just close your eyes become this image. Pretend it has already happened – how good do you look? How good do you feel? Daydream now.

That's the first of many times I am going to ask you to close your eyes and picture or feel something, so if you haven't done it shame on you! You must DO this book not just read it. This programme is tried and tested, it has worked for many people, but you must take responsibility for making this programme work for YOU.

Now imagine yourself again, enjoying the process of change, recognise it is painful to go back to where you were before and pleasurable to continue along in the direction you have chosen. There is no hurdle; there is nothing in the way of you and your goal, only pleasure. Believe it or not the nutrition side is the least important aspect of what you need to change to lose weight. There is a two week programme in this book that will give you a great start so you see results straight away, with some great long term guidelines and a structure to change how and what you eat: but changing the way you think and feel about yourself and how you "use" food is the only way to achieve the shape and size you desire – permanently. What this book is not, is a diet, there are NO foods that are forbidden! There's NOTHING YOU CAN'T HAVE, but there is one very important golden rule that must never ever be broken and it's this:

If you don't enjoy it – don't eat it!

New techiques for a New You!

In this book you will find a mixture of techniques for you to *change your mind* about how you eat, including TFT (Thought Field Therapy), NLP (Neuro Linguistic Programming), Self Hypnosis and Life Coaching. All of these work together to empower *you* so you can achieve what you desire. This is not a book you read. It's a book you do! Just Do It Now.

DO YOU CHOOSE PLEASURE OR PAIN?

Sit for a moment and think about all the painful things you associate with being fat. Such as things you can't do, or how you feel about yourself. Using the arrow on page 8, write all these things at the "PAIN" end. Ask your unconscious mind to fully associate pain with not changing and staying as you are now.

Next think about all the things that will be different when you have changed and are slimmer, how you will feel, things you CAN do. Write these at the PLEASURE end. Ask your unconscious mind to fully associate PLEASURE into changing so you CAN feel and experience all these things.

Take a good look at this worksheet every night or at least once during the day for at least two weeks, and you will begin to programme your mind to associate pain with not changing and pleasure in doing all the new behaviours you are going to learn from the WLIM system.

PLEASURE

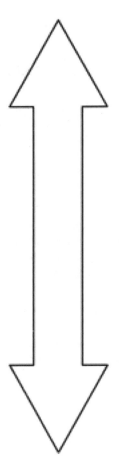

PAIN

START HERE...

Read this exercise through, then close your eyes and allow yourself to daydream as you reflect on what you need to do:

Remember a time in your life when something wonderful happened, such as the birth of a child, meeting the partner of your dreams, or a time when your parents made you feel really fantastic about something you did or said, it may be a fleeting moment you had or a place you visited, anything that you can recall in detail that made you deliciously happy. When you have decided on a moment close your eyes and go back in time and re-experience that moment, see everything you saw then but as if time had stood still so you can take as long to look at things as you need to, hear the sounds around you, voices, background noises, anything you could hear at the time. Then remember how it actually felt and put that feeling back on, as if it were a garment and wear it as you look around and listen. Spend a few minutes re-living and re-experiencing the moment in every sense. Notice HOW you experience this memory; are you making still pictures? Running a movie? Is there sound? Does it stimulate a feeling in your body – if so where? Your stomach? Your chest? Be aware of exactly HOW you are processing this memory.

We will come back to your memory throughout this chapter: Its not so much what the memory is, but *how* you remembered it that is important: understanding your unique pattern, the way that you process important information is the key to bringing about change.

As we go about our lives we are taking in massive amounts of information, if you were to walk down a supermarket aisle now, your brain would be processing all the information received from your eyes and ears, every label on every packet, every colour of every fruit and the sound of everyone talking and moving. If you were to retain all this information you wouldn't be able to access what you needed quickly, so much of it is deleted, the rest is filtered out through three different systems and stored in your brains hard drive, where you can access it quickly whenever you need to. You use all three filters all the time, but you will probably have an order of preference or importance, so that information delivered to you through your primary filter will have more of an impact.

Take a moment and now think about drinking a cup of deliciously flavoured perculated coffee (if you don't like coffee use tea, hot chocolate or any other similar drink): What is the experience like for you? Do you picture a mug of steaming coffee? See yourself in a particular place drinking it? Do you hear the sound of the percolator bubbling and hissing? Do you remember the warm feeling as the coffee goes down? Or the smell? Or just how you feel after a great cup of coffee?

In reality you use all three filters to some extent all the time, but you will probably have a preference. If someone wants to influence you, and they understand how you receive and process information, it makes it easier for them to get their message across in a way you are likely to react positively to. In our personal lives we tend to mix with people who have a similar way of processing information to us. If you think about your closest friends, they probably "see the world as you do", come to the same conclusions about things during discussions, i.e. "feel the same way". When you are with people "on your wavelength" you have natural rapport.

Think about your happy memory. Bearing in mind the three filters, Visual Audio Kinaesthetic, (VAK) put in order how you recalled your happy moments. Did you see the images before you got the feeling, or the other way around, or did the sounds come back to you first? Think carefully and rank the 3 filters in order.

VISUAL

This means you think in pictures, if you immediately see the cup and the steam coming from it, and you literally see yourself drinking the coffee, then you are using visual filters.

Characteristics of Visual Thinkers:
- speak quickly using visual words, eg. "look, see"
- have rapid shallow breathing
- when speaking make arm gestures in the air to "create" the image they see
- often show their tension in their physical posture

AUDITORY

If you heard the sound of the peculator bubbling and hissing away, or the sounds in the room where the coffee was made then sounds are important to you, you are using auditory filters.

Characteristics of Auditory thinkers:
- speak in a rhythmical or tuneful manner using words like 'sounds' and 'hear'
- talk mid tone
- breathe mid chest
- use lower arm gestures when speaking

FEELINGS (KINESTHETIC)

If you get a warm feeling, can remember the smell or taste of good coffee and recall the experience of drinking it before you see or hear things you are using kinesthetic filters.

Characteristics of a Feelings thinker:
- speak in a resonant low tone using words like 'feel', 'sense'
- breath low and slowly in the chest
- when speaking gesture low and to the right
- have laid back posture

1.

2.

3.

All this information is processed in a pattern or code that is specific to you, someone else with the same information may have a completely different thought process and create a completely different memory pattern from you, even if you have both had what seemed to be the exact same experience.

Understanding this is important because it shows you how exposed you are to certain suggestions. The people who know most about this process are usually involved in advertising or sales. Millions of pounds is spent identifying different groups of people who might want to purchase a particular item and how they are likely to respond to a specific filter. Let me give you an example: A couple of years ago a new mobile phone company launched with one of the most successful campaigns ever seen. It involved "images" of communications, such as a wife at home in her dressing gown and slippers, ready for bed, a separate shot of her husband working away in the arctic taking measurements in the snow, all wrapped up in a fur coat and gloves – clearly miles away from her. In the advert we see her step out of the house, walk across the snow in her slippers, right up to her husband and plant a goodnight kiss on his cheek. He stands and smiles – but she's not there. Then it becomes clear this image represents a text she has sent wishing him goodnight and sending him a kiss. The primary filter for this advert is the *feeling* of closeness you can get by sending a text to someone who is far away, but they used powerful *visual* images to get that feeling across. There was a whole range of adverts for

"Orange" and not one of them showed a phone. They all showed a "feeling" you could get from using a mobile phone.

Everything we do is based on how we want to feel. Do we buy chocolate because of how it looks? If the adverts for chocolate associated it with a horrible feeling, instead of the luscious indulgent feelings they portray, and they made it look disgusting, do you think they would sell so much chocolate? Certainly not. Imagine an advert showing someone looking repulsive, covered in filth and scabs and looking angry and miserable eating mouldy looking chocolate, it's not so appealing when it doesn't represent something you want to feel yourself.

Feelings, such as feeling sexy, indulgent, or just plain feeling good are used to sell us unhealthy products every single day.

When it comes to food, the feelings we associate with specific items determine how much of it and when we eat it. Think now of a food you think you "shouldn't" have, but you regularly eat, what feeling do you associate with that food? If you didn't get that good feeling when you ate it, if it gave you an unpleasant feeling, would you still want it? How often do you eat just to get a feeling other than to satisfy genuine hunger? If you are fatter than you would like, then probably quite often.

Being "In State"

All three filters are working all the time, but when you are "in state" the receptors in your brain are more efficient and you take in more information in more detail than you otherwise would for everyday mundane things. There are peak states that are both good and bad, for example if the love of your life asks you to spend the rest of your life with them you are likely to be in a good peak state! Conversely if someone you love dies your intense sense of grief is bad peak state. On both occasions memories of these events are incredibly vivid, you can recount in minute detail things you wouldn't otherwise have noticed. In the case of good peak state this is an advantage, but in the case of bad peak state it can bring back an intensity of pain you would rather not remember.

We can apply this to the earlier concept of pleasure and pain, the more intense the pain you associate with previous diets, i.e. the more "in state" you are when you think about it, the less likely you are to succeed in future diets. You can become very negative whenever you think about dieting. In TFT terms this is "Psychological Reversal" or PR, which will almost certainly block your ability to change your behaviour. In practical terms it means you are very negative when it comes to "dieting" and you will actually sabotage your own behaviour. There is a simple and easy technique to correct this negativity later in the book.

Some NLP techniques combined with a generous helping of common sense, can help you remove the pain altogether i.e. take out anything and everything negative that you did whilst dieting that you didn't like. Some of this you can do by yourself now, simply by deciding not to eat foods you don't like just because they are "slimming". NO MORE DIET FOOD!
Overeating is a way of covering up a negative feeling, usually anxiety. We don't like the feeling we have so we eat to replace it with something else. Remove the anxiety and theres no need to overeat. This is where TFT comes in.

Patterns between feelings and food can be set from a very early age. If as a child whenever you were upset your mum said "stop crying and you can have a biscuit" or "if you are good you can have a biscuit/piece of cake" you take these associations of eating to feel better and using food as a reward into your adult life. Subconsciously they influence your food choices for as long as you let them. If when you were a child your mum had said every-time you were upset, "stop crying and I will take you to the park and we will play with a ball" and you spent many happy hours throwing a ball around, as an adult when you are upset you are more likely to go out and kick a few balls around whenever you want to feel better, rather than grab a biscuit.

Your brain is like a computer hard drive, and each time you see, hear or feel something this information is entered onto the computer and it does a search, it matches it with either the same experience or a similar one that you have had before i.e. a memory pattern and automatically replays the same response you had then. If you had a bad experience on your first ever flight, and the plane went through rough weather and turbulence and you experienced new sensations you didn't like that made you afraid – that would create a "memory file" in your brain. The next time you got on a plane you would be likely to feel the same sensations even if the weather was good and flying conditions were smooth, it is likely you would still "remember" to feel afraid.

The first step in overcoming this type of reaction is to recognise the patterns when they occur, once you have identified them you can change them. If you feel fed up or depressed or even bored and would normally reach for the chocolate automatically, but instead use TFT to eliminate the anxiety and correct the Psychological Reversal, (I will show you how to do both of these a little later in the book), then the instinct or craving is eliminated. Then indulge in something pleasurable that does not involve food, like a long relaxing bath with candles and plenty of soapy suds with your favourite music playing in the background, or shut yourself away from the world and get lost in your favourite book, or put some headphones on and listen to your favourite CD, or anything that gives you space and time to put yourself in a different state, after a just a few repetitions your instinctive behaviour when you feel negative, will change from turning to food for comfort, to indulging in something other than chocolate that you can enjoy without any negative side effects (i.e. fat gain!").

I have included two 'Craving Crusher' exercises so you can stop negative food cravings. I will show you how to do these shortly and you can use them with any food you want to give up. First let me give you an example of how easy it is to "anchor" the desire for food: I often travel to Spain and got to know the local area well. One of my favourite restaurants is owned by a Spanish guy named Tony, and we have it off to a fine art that we take the same flight each time which arrives about 1.30 pm and go straight to Tony's for a delicious and slightly boozy long lunch in the sunshine. A perfect way to start a holiday! Because we know we are going to have a big lunch I have a very light breakfast in anticipation and to "make room!" On one occasion recently the flight was running late, and by the time we boarded I was so hungry I felt ill. Sitting in my seat I heard the clink of the steward coming around with the trolley for drinks and snacks, I was very hungry and really wanted something and I needed it NOW! I should tell you at this point that I have a slight intolerance to wheat, and some breads in particular cause me to bloat and give me extremely bad wind! Not recommended for flying as the poor people next to me, in-front and behind have nowhere to escape. When I asked the steward what he had to eat is was between bread and chocolate, so it had to be chocolate and I had a can of Coke to go with it. My peak state was quite high because I was very exited about the holiday, and also because I was frustrated at not leaving on time. I ate it in seconds, infact I ate so quickly I barely tasted what I was eating. I didn't stop and "think" about what it was or even how it tasted.

We had a lovely break, and on the way home I was sitting in my seat on the plane when I heard the clink- clink of the trolley and was immediately transported back in my mind to the flight out, the steward asked if I would like anything – without thinking I said "yes please a bar of chocolate and a coke" as I was eating it I thought "why did I have this, I am not even hungry?" and realised that even just that one time on the flight out, had been enough to make a memory pattern or association that if you have chocolate and coke on a plane you feel better.

Next time we travelled I took a CD player and played my favourite CD when the trolley came round, so I didn't hear it and was able to break the pattern. It would have been so easy to fall into the chocolate trap and do the same again. It's all about choosing how you react. We are making new patterns all the time as our brains are constantly trying to match experiences we have with previous experiences to tell us how we should feel and what we should do. A common trait for people who are fat, is to eat quickly without actually thinking about what they are eating. Ironically they think about food most of the time when they are not eating.

All behaviour is a result of "state", which is just another way of describing how you feel. Have you ever felt "in a terrible state" or how about "a state of ecstasy"? Each state brings about a different set of responses and behaviours.

The most effective way to change your state is to associate fully into a different image: When you think about something you are either using associated thinking or disassociated thinking:

DISASSOCIATED THINKING	ASSOCIATED THINKING
Thinking about something from outside of your body, seeing it from an observers eyes and watching how you/other people react without actually experiencing the feeling yourself, you are merely a spectator	Thinking about something as if you were inside your body experiencing it, seeing it through your eyes and feeling what you would be feeling if you were there. You imagine having the experience yourself.

A critical part of learning is to recognise that your brain does not know the difference between an imagined experience and a real life experience. If you imagine something vividly enough in a fully associated state, then it actually happens as a real experience as far as your brain is concerned and you create a memory pattern which you automatically revert to every time you are in the same situation.

Have you ever been thinking or worrying about something bad that *might happen,* where you felt so upset/worried/nervous that you felt physically sick and your mind was in a whirl,-- your heart rate increased, breathing increased and you felt physically as well as emotionally terrible? Even though nothing had actually happened, in your mind and body it felt as if it had. Am I right?

When I was married, my ex-husband was in the fire-brigade: If he was late home from work, I would stand at the window waiting visualising him struggling for breath in some inferno risking life and limb. I would feel physically sick with worry, in fact in my mind he really was in an inferno, so when he did come home I was in such a peak state I almost collapsed with relief when he walked in the door. He was a fireman for seven years and I never learnt to handle it because I didn't know then how to change my thinking. Time after time I would stand at the window "doing" worry, I had a great strategy, being a visual thinker I started with a movie of a terrible fire and the building collapsing with him in it, the other guys on his shift trying in vain to pull him out and then debating who should come and tell me the awful news, then I pictured a senior fireman walking up my drive and knocking on my door with his hat under his arm saying "Mrs Thomson, I think you need to sit down" then I ran the conversation in my head, even to the extent of the conversation I would have to have with his mum when I called her to tell her the awful news, as this was going on I developed a heavy "black" feeling deep in the pit of my stomach, sometimes I was actually physically sick and almost always had to rush to the loo to empty my bowels as the feeling deepened. As you can see I had an excellent strategy for "doing" worry. By imagining terrible things that didn't actually happen I became psychologically reversed and very anxious. In my mind it was totally real, even though I knew consciously it was all "in my mind".

In terms of learning new behaviours this process of accepting imagined events as real can be useful: if you imagine yourself doing something really well over and over again, your brain thinks you have really done it well and a new positive pattern or skill can be established.

Some research shows it takes us up to twenty one times of repeating a new pattern for it to overwrite the old one. This is fine if you want to use "will power", that is deny yourself what you want twenty one times and replace it with something else that's not really what you want. If you do that in a reversed (PR) or negative state of mind then the chances are it won't work anyway, but if you do it in a powerfully associated state and you associate **pleasure** with the new pattern and **pain** with not changing, then your brain will respond quickly and effectively. TFT can change your state from negative to positive in seconds and some NLP techniques for changing patterns need only be done once to be effective. Change can be immediate. The more you believe it is working the quicker it works. Do not believe it when people tell you it takes weeks, months or even years to change. Just because they just don't know how to do it faster, doesn't mean you cant *change right now,* and I will show you how.

When you watch the World Championships or Olympics in any sport you will see the athletes mentally going through their performance or event before they start. This vital preparation means they have already run the race or completed the event with perfect technique, this makes it easier to access the memory file and repeat the same techniques when doing it for real. When Shaun Murphy won the World Snooker Championships at Sheffield in April 2005, it was the first time he had ever reached a major final. Even for regular snooker spectators he was relatively unknown: the arena at Sheffield is famous for its atmosphere, it's almost tangible, the players are so close to the spectators they can almost touch them. There is not really enough space in the arena at all, to quote a former World Champion John Parrott speaking about the auditorium "its total is greater than the sum of its parts". Many world class players crumble when they experience it and cannot cope with the pressure. When interviewed after winning the final the presenter asked Shaun "How did you cope so well being in the final for the first time here at the Crucible" to which he replied "Oh no I have been here hundreds of times", He wasn't in the final for the first time, in his mind he had already played and won it many times. He had "designed" his programme so well that when he got there he already knew exactly what he had to do. If you have the complete WLIM system, use CD1 'Making Changes' now. See audio information sheet at the back for more details.

This simple yet powerful technique can help you in numerous situations, for example if you want to pass a driving test: for the few days prior to your test you get not only practical practice i.e. in a car, you also sit and vividly image yourself doing every single manoeuvre perfectly, providing you have been taught properly and your mental practice is perfect, you will set a memory pattern that is easy to re-access. I remember from my gymnastic training as a teenager if I was learning a new move and did it wrong once, I often found myself making the same mistake over and over again. My coach used to remind us "only perfect practice makes perfect" so if you practice (real or imagined) doing something badly you will become very good at doing it badly! In simple terms if you "see yourself" failing at something then you are showing your brain how to fail. People who think of failure often become very good at it. It's not just about being optimistic, it's about planning and preparing your brain, in combination with a good strategy, to get the result you want, whether its for you to change what you eat or learn any other new skill you need.

Using your filters (VAK) you can change how and where you file information in your brain: instead of filing something you like eating under "pleasure", you can change your response and file it under "pain", so that you no longer want or desire that particular food. Have you ever eaten (or drunk!) something that made you ill, and since then you have never been able to touch it without feeling sick? This is because the way your brain is wired to respond to that particular food changes when have a violent reaction to it, so even the thought of it can make you feel sick. The food itself doesn't change, but how you feel about it does. A few years ago I was on a dolphin watching trip in Florida and they gave us a ham and cheese roll, which combined with the rocking motion of the boat made me violently ill. Since then I cannot even think about a ham and cheese sandwich without my throat tightening at the thought. I had to stop eating it – ever.

You can use this "Craving Crushing" technique to stop yourself wanting foods that make you fat and unhealthy. When you re-wire your brain so that the thought of chocolate makes you feel ill, it's not painful to give it up – it's painful *not* to give it up! This is the first of two powerful craving crushing techniques I am going to show you now that you can use to change what you want to eat.

CRAVING CRUSHER (1)

Its not enough to just read this – you have to DO this exercise

Read each step before you do it, when you have completed it move onto the next step.

If you would like to change the way you think about a specific unhealthy food then read on. This classic NLP technique requires you to get TOTALLY into peak state with every taste or experience I ask of you. Remember this type of technique works because your brain does not know the difference between a real experience and a (vividly) imaged one so be as vivid as possible! Read each step thoroughly FIRST, then do it in a fully associated state, actually be there and get your taste buds and sense of smell finely tuned for action. It's important to complete each stage fully before you move on, there's no time limit, it takes most people approximately five to ten minutes. Bearing in mind the brain learns fast, once you understand what to do – do it fast. If it helps then do it with a friend, both read through the exercise first so you are confident and then take turns to read out the instructions (one at a time) to each other and take each other through each phase.

Step 1. Tap the side of your hand (karate spot) 15-20 times (see picture pg 28)

Step 2 Visualise whatever food you want to lose your desire for: be very specific, you cannot do it by imagining a group of foods, it has to be an individual item. Hold that image and be aware of all the sensations or feelings you associate with it. Imagine you are putting it into your mouth, feel the texture of the food as it begins to melt in your mouth, feel it coat your tongue and your teeth. You may run your tongue over your teeth to really feel, it taste it and smell it.

Step 3. Now think about a food you cannot stand, something that TOTALLY repulses you. If theres something that has made you physically sick in the past then go with that, the more repulsive it makes you feel the better. Imagine this food is in your mouth now, double how disgusting it is, imagine it contains a few maggots or pubic hairs to make it even more repulsive. Feel the texture as it sticks to your mouth holding that horrid taste and sensation. Give it a rancid or equally unpleasant smell. Squeeze the finger and thumb on your left hand together to "anchor" that revulsion to a physical action. Break the thought pattern for a few seconds, imagine a blank white screen, then resume the repulsion exercise. When it gets absolutely intolerable and you feel sick for real when you think about the food, squeeze the finger and thumb on the left hand. Do this at least 5 times until everytime you squeeze that finger and thumb you remember to remember how gross the taste of this food is.

Step 4. Now think about the food you want to give up and imagine it combined with the "bad" food you have just anchored. Really mix up the tastes and textures until you can no longer think about the original food without combining it with an overpowering taste of the food you hate – it's as if they are both in your mouth now. When they are inextricably mixed, imagine eating both foods bound together and although you can taste the original "nice" food, it is overwhelmed by the disgusting and repulsive sensations of taste and smell of the repulsive food. As you do this, squeeze the finger and thumb on the left hand. Break your thought and repeat at least 5 times, each time imagining the taste gets worse. Do this until you are actually retching or heaving when you imagine eating the foods forever combined together. File this revolting taste and memory of this food as "disgusting" in your mind.

Step 5. To finish off and finalise, sit still and visualise your now repulsive food way ahead in-front of you but massive in size, as big as a wall, and notice there is a piece of elastic stretching between you and it, pulled really tightly. In a moment after I count to three, that elastic will snap and the food will zoom towards you like a missile, just as its about to smash into your face you will notice the foul smell and image, it will make a horrid sound that only you will recognise as being a sound you hate, perhaps a screech or the sound of a nail on a blackboard - make it the worst sound you have ever heard and allow all the horrid sensations to flood into your mind and through your body, then very quickly imagine this wall of revolting food passing right through your body, mixing the horrid taste smell and sound together, until it is totally behind you. Now this whole process takes only a couple of seconds but your senses are at their peak so make it intense, actually feel it go through you. Are you ready? Can you see the food? Can you sense the smells and the foul taste of it mixed with vomit that's about to come flying towards you? When you can, complete this final stage...

Get ready ...... one....two....three...... slam! push through and the food is behind you and gone.

Tap To Stop Overeating

Food addicts vary from those who constantly overeat, to those who overeat very specifically on a specific food or at a specific time – usually the same time each day. Food addiction is like any addiction, whether it's to drugs or gambling, you started to do it because you liked the feeling you got when you did it, you had some negative emotion or state you didn't like and you saw food as a way to make you feel better. When it worked the first time, the new behaviour then became anchored to making you feel better, to "cheering you up". It reinforced a wrongly held belief that overeating made you feel good. Any addict cannot just stop the behaviour with will-power, they need to eliminate the reason for the addiction. TFT can do this quickly and effectively. This is the first of several TFT algorithms I will teach you.

All TFT points are located on meridian pathways. Unlike acupuncture which is invasive in that it pierces the skin and you cannot do it yourself, TFT requires only that you tap each spot gently, just firmly enough to put energy into the system. You can do it easily yourself. Points must be tapped in a specific order or pattern called an algorithm. There are various algorithms for different psychological emotions, such as anxiety, anger, frustration etc. However what matters most is that you MUST be thinking very specifically about the problem when you tap. For example this algorithm for food craving is the same as the algorithm for anxiety, but the thought field is totally different. If you are thinking about your car whilst tapping to eliminate a food craving it simply will not work. You have to be IN the exact thought field, actually experiencing the emotion you want to eliminate. In that way the same or similar algorithm may be used to eliminate a variety of negative emotions.

All the treatment points are listed below for future reference to be used in other algorithms. Not all points are used for each treatment. Once you have identified and practiced gently tapping on the points then read the "protocol". This protocol is exactly the same for each algorithm.

Tapping treatment points chart

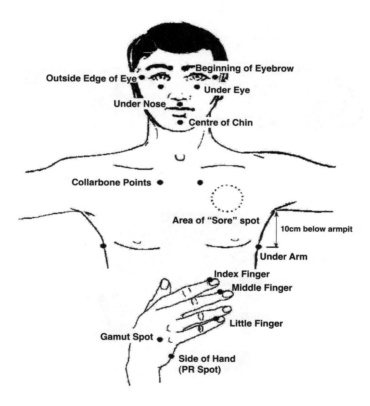

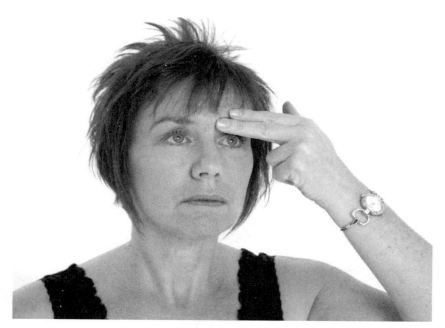

Eyebrow (eb)

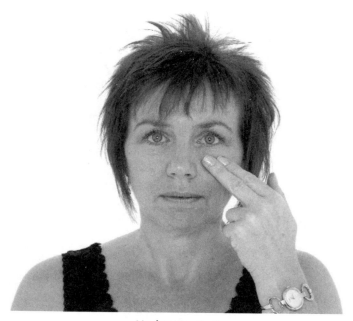

Under eye (ue)

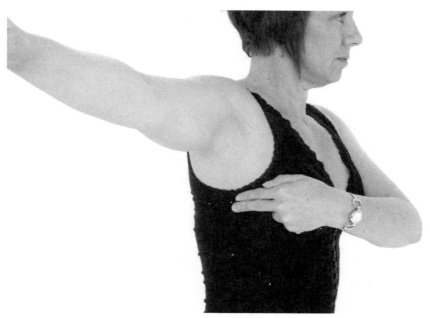

Under arm (ua)

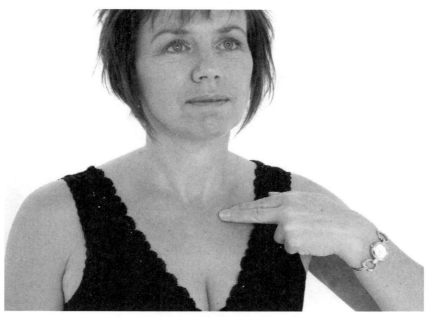

Collar bone (cb)

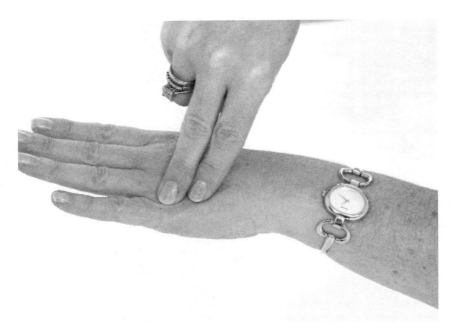

Gamut spot (g)

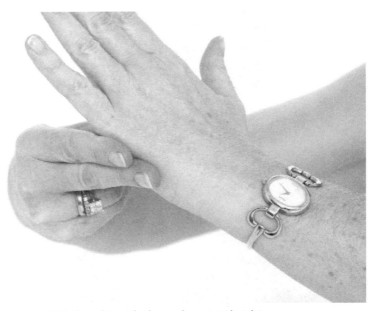

Side hand/psychological reversal (sh)
Karate spot

Tapping Protocol

Each treatment follows the same pattern:

1. Focus your thought on the "problem". Ensure you stay in this thought the entire time. Rate the problem between 1-10 with 10 being terrible and 1 being no problem. This is called a SUD (subjective unit of distress) and is important to measure your progress.

2. Gently tap each of the designated points in the stated order (algorithm) 10–15 times, hard enough to put energy into the system but not hard enough to hurt.

3. Tap the top of the hand in-between the small and ring finger knuckle continually, (either hand) this is the Gamut spot (see pg 28). Whilst tapping do the following: keeping the head still move the eyes only – Close then open the eyes (slow blink), then look

    - Down left (pg 31)

    - Down right (pg 31)

    - Circle the eyes 360° one way (as if looking at all the numbers on a clock face)

    - Circle the eyes 360° the other way around

    - Hum out loud a few bars

    - Count out loud 1 2 3 4 5

    - Hum out loud a few bars

    This is called 9g

4.   Repeat the original tapping sequence (algorithm)

5.   Take a new SUD. If the problem is less repeat the treatment. It may take several "rounds" but if the SUD goes down 2 or more points each time it is working. Repeat until the negative emotion, is eliminated

6.   When SUD is 2 or less, tap the gamut spot continually and keeping the head still, look down into your cheekbones and SLOWLY roll the eyes upwards, first to look straight ahead then continue upwards until you are looking into or under your eyebrows.

If the SUD is still the same, or sticks at any point during the treatment tap the side of the hand, then rub the sore spot just under the left collar bone, then tap under the nose and start the process again from the beginning.

Craving Crusher (2)

First either place in front of you or strongly visualise and think about the food you crave. Take a SUD, i.e. if before the treatment you would "kill" for a bar of chocolate (or whatever the food is) that would be a 10, and a 1 = no desire for the food at all. Repeat the treatment until the craving has gone and SUD is a 1.

There are three algorithms that eliminate cravings and addictive urges, try each of them whilst focusing on your desire for the food and see which works best for you. You may find one algorithm works better for one food and another for another. This can also be an effective technique to stop the desire for cigarettes and is a vital part of my "stop smoking" therapy. Use it if you smoke or on friends that smoke and see for yourself.

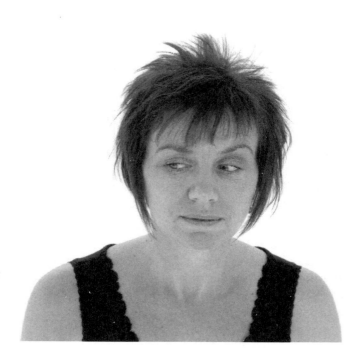

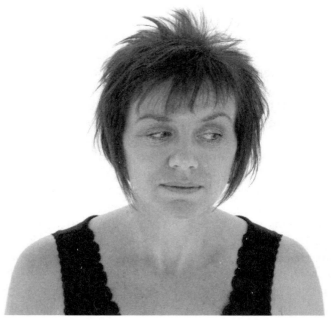

9g

Algorithm 1	Algorithm 2	Algorithm 3
Side hand (karate spot)	Side hand (karate spot)	Side hand (karate spot)
	Under eyes	Under arm
Collar bones	Collar bones	Under eye
Under eyes	Under arm	Collar bone
Collar bones	Collar bones	9g
9g	9g	Repeat tapping
Repeat tapping	Repeat tapping	

This treatment is quick, easy and effective. Learn it well so that you can "tap" whenever you have a food craving to make it vanish. It takes little over a minute, sometimes just seconds. If you consider the saying "a minute on the lips a lifetime on the hips" it is certainly time well spent.

❖   ❖   ❖

After you lay down a new memory pattern, there is often a feeling of confusion, or feeling slightly muddled, this is a good sign! It means your brain is re-wiring and undoing the previous pattern. I once heard it described like the scene in Harry Potter, where the staircases in Hogwarts move as you stand on them and you are not quite sure where you are going, but its not where you thought you were going!

Elephants are a good example of how powerful a memory pattern can be: when they are small they are chained to a post so they cannot go out of their enclosure. They learn that this connection stops them from moving outside of a designated area. As they get older these chains are replaced with rope and eventually sometimes just string. The elephant doesn't try to see if he can break it by going too far, all the time he is attached to any kind of rope or chain his memory pattern tells him he cannot get past the end of the rope/string so he doesn't try. The elephant never forgets the string limits how far he can travel. In reality he could walk away and break the string – but he doesn't because he doesn't believe he can.

CHANGE YOUR BEHAVIOUR...
AND BE IN CONTROL

At the moment you want to change something specific in your life, i.e. your weight or shape. You have had enough of being fat. Very soon you will have all the strategies you need to change whatever you want, not just your weight but ANYTHING you are unhappy with in your life. All the answers to everything you want to change are out there, they may not yet be in your head where they will be, but they are "out there". Once you get them in your head you will be immensely powerful, in fact you will be formidable. You will have the POWER TO CHANGE anything you want.

Many people think willpower is the answer, as we have already discovered willpower is a painful and ineffective way to try and change something, so here's the good news *no more will power is required!* What *is* required is a new set of strategies, in terms of how you think, behave and react – the choices you make. Motivation is also a useful tool, it gets you started (you are naturally motivated to avoid pain as we have already discovered) yet even the most motivated person will not succeed without a strategy. To quote Anthony Robbins "If you want to see a sunset, no matter how hard or fast you run – if you run East it will never happen." That's why this book is so different and unique, I am giving you all the information you need, and motivating you, but I am also giving you an effective mental *and* nutrition strategy. Either one without the other is not enough, you need both. There are some excellent self help or NLP based books out there for weight loss, and also some excellent "diets" but the reality is you need to think every day and you need to eat everyday, so lets put the two together and get the job done. This is what you need.

Programme your brain to do what *YOU* want to do, otherwise other people will programme you to do what they want you to do!

Your view of your past, the way you have processed information and your memories and associations dictate your behaviour today. These memory files can limit your ability to see your future as a place full of possibilities and different choices. In the film "The Matrix" Neo can simply "plug in" to the computer and learn and install any new skill or behaviour he needs. He learnt several martial arts after a few hours of IN MIND PROGRAMMING.

If you had a bump on the head and in a split second all your current learned behaviours disappeared and you had the chance to re-programme everything you have ever learnt, what behaviours or new habits would you install instead? What effect would that have on your life, on how you feel, on what you achieve? If you knew you couldn't fail what would you do?

Exercise

Spend at least five minutes now doing just that, sit back, close your eyes and imagine how you would like to be programmed. See hear and feel yourself reacting to things as you would if, you have already installed these new programmes. Be *disassociated* i.e. imagine you are watching yourself. Start with a typical week day, what will you do when you wake up? What will you eat? Go through the entire day watching yourself, seeing yourself with these new behaviours and habits that result in a slimmer, healthier, happier you. Then do the same for a weekend or a non work day. Then watch yourself on a night out with friends, maybe going out for a meal. What can you see yourself doing differently to what you did before? When you are happy that you can see yourself doing everything you need to do, having the body you want, being happy with the way you are going about it, actually imagine yourself inside that body. Watch the same movie but this time be *associated,* i.e. be inside your body and watch thorough your eyes as you go through your day. Step "inside "you" and start the movie again.

Now you have made this visualisation into a movie and watch it regularly. Make time each day, for either just a couple of minutes daydreaming or create a few thoughts and images before you go to sleep, and run them over and over again until the images are so familiar and comfortable they become automatic. Remember to remember what you see.

You are intelligent, you know how you got fat: Think about it now honestly. Then write down the 3 things you did most often that made you fat.

Fat behaviours

1.

2

3

Now think about what the exact opposite behaviours are, so if one is "I eat more than I need" then the opposite would be "I control my portion sizes, I stop *before* I overeat". Another might be "I sit down at every opportunity" the opposite would be "I move about whenever I can, I am more active". It's all basic stuff and requires only common sense, not a sports science degree! Now you have three new behaviour patterns that guarantee a new slim you. These are the first of many changes you can make now you have the skills.

New Behaviours that will make me slim

1

2

3

So now to the question you do not want to hear – what has been stopping you from changing these behaviours? Look at them one at a time, read the behaviour and then ask yourself what would happen if you *change it right now?*

The reason you ran the "fat" programmes is that you wrongly perceived it would be too painful to change them, even though you are unhappy with the way you look and feel because of them. It goes back to the fundamental principle of PLEASURE vs PAIN. You wrongly associated pleasure with overeating, when in fact it is uncomfortable and unpleasant. It is possible to change these fat behaviours – you simply need to associate intense pain with them, and associate immense pleasure with deleting them and replacing them with new ones. You also need to check for psychological reversal (PR) over your desire to lose weight. Let me explain.

Psychological Reversal (PR)
Your body has a polarity, it's overall polarity can be either positive or negative, and it's constantly changing from one to the other. When its negative it is termed "reversal". There are different levels of reversal, all of which affect your mood, the way you think and behave and to a large extent your heath. In this next section I will show you how easy it is to correct these reversals. In a recent interview Dr Callahan was discussing his discoveries and the subsequent creation of TFT: he said that of all his findings, the most significant was identifying Psychological Reversal and learning how to correct it.

When you are in positive polarity you feel better, you make

better decisions, you learn better and your body can heal better. When you are negative you are more likely to make mistakes, turn left instead of right, put the milk in the oven and the pie in the fridge, may forget even simple things, be negative and self defeatist or even depressed. Physiologically your body will be less efficient at healing when your polarity is negative.

Diffferent Levels of Reversal

Global or Massive Reversal
If you are massively reversed it affects you psychologically in anything and everything you do say and think. It also affects your body's physiology.

Specific Reversal
Commonly people are reversed in one specific area or thought. For example many of my clients are successful in all other areas of their life, except weight loss. They have achieved great academic, professional and personal success and the only thing they ever "fail" at is weight loss. This is because they have a specific PR to losing weight. Luckily this can be easily corrected using the most simple of TFT techniques and takes just a few seconds every day.

The best way to test for PR is using applied kinesiology. You will need someone to help you test.

The following techniques have their basis in TFT, however based on my extensive experience in this field.I have adapted certain aspects of the process to enable you to get the best possible weight loss results without me actually being with you.

1.   Stand upright and place one arm out directly to the side. With your other arm place the hand over the head (but not touching) with the palm facing downwards. Have your partner press firmly down on your arm as you resist and hold your arm still. Notice how strong you feel and the exact effort it takes you to resist. You need to assess just how much pressure you both need to exert for your arm to stay in the same position. If your partner is much stronger than you, do not allow them to press

so hard your arm collapses. Between the two of you work out how hard you have to resist to keep the arm in the same position and how much pressure they can exert until just before your arm drops. It is important your partner exerts a constant pressure, for about 3-4 seconds, without bouncing. They press, you resist.

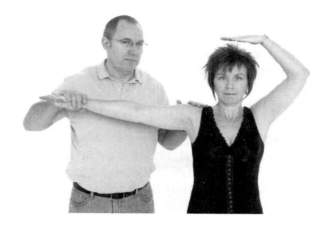

Strong arm

2.   Now turn your hand over so the back of your hand is facing your head and the palm is facing up. Have your partner exert the same amount of pressure as before and resist.

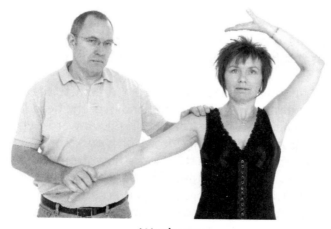

Weak arm

You will probably notice a drastic difference between the two, i.e. with your palm facing your head your arm is strong, as this has positive polarity, and when you flip over so the back of your hand is facing your head, your arm is weak, as this has negative polarity.

If both are the same strength, or it is the wrong way round i.e. palm down is weak and palm up strong, it indicates a massive PR and you need to tap the side of your hand 15-20 times and repeat the exercise. This technique is reliable for almost everyone. Occasionally someone cannot feel a difference and this indicates the presence of toxins, which is discussed later in the book and can be identified and corrected using TFT Voice Technology.

Once you have identified a clear difference so that palm down is strong and palm up is weak, you can use muscle testing to ask your body and your "unconscious" mind questions. You only need to use one arm once you have tested for reversal.

Place your arm out to the side, have your partner apply the same pressure for 3-4 secs and say "My name is ..." say your correct name as you resist and notice how strong your arm is. Rest for a few seconds then repeat, but this time say "My name is daffy duck" and with your partner exerting the same pressure notice how weak your arm becomes in comparison to when you are telling the truth.

Once you are confident with the process, use it to test the

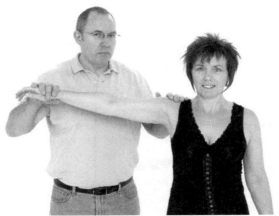

Strong arm – correct name

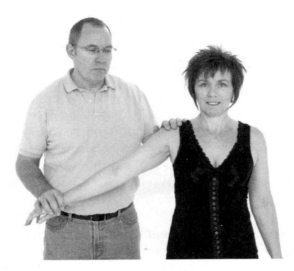

Weak arm = Daffy Duck

statements in the table below, whilst focusing on your desired weight. (It's important to stay in the thought field throughout the test.)

Statement	Strong arm	Weak arm
I want to lose weight	You genuinely want to lose weight and are likely to be successful	On a deeper level you do not want to and will sabotage your own attempts to lose weight *Step 1* *Tap the side of your hand 15-20 times* *If arm is still weak on statement see corrective treatment*
I want to stay overweight	On a deeper level you do not want to lose weight and will sabotage your own attempts to lose weight **Step 1** *Tap the side of your hand 15-20 times* *If arm is still weak on statement see corrective treatment*	You genuinely want to lose weight and are likely to be successful

Corrective Treatment

1.   Gently rub the sore spot under the left collar bone in circular motions for about 20-30 seconds, then tap under your nose 15-20 times (see pg 25).

Repeat the muscle test. *If you still get a weak arm when you say "I want to lose weight" then move to step 2*

2.   Tap the side of the hand continuously and repeat the following affirmations whilst focusing on wanting to lose weight

"I want to be over this problem"
"I want to be completely over this problem"
"I will be over this problem"
"I will be completely over this problem"
"I want to be even better"

Tap under your nose and repeat the above affirmations

Repeat the muscle test with the statement "I want to lose weight". In most cases this will clear the reversal.

I recommend as part of your programme, each morning you tap the side of your hand whilst thinking about your desired weight and repeat the affirmations whilst focusing on your desired weight and shape.

The great thing about TFT is its very effective and has ABSOLUTELY NO side effects. It takes no more than a minute and can be done anywhere anytime. Even without the affirmations, tapping the side of your hand regularly throughout the day whilst thinking about your desired weight, will help keep you positive and on track and help control overeating and craving.

Collarbone Breathing (CB2)

In addition to tapping regularly for PR throughout the day there is another exercise that takes approximately 2 minutes and is vital for achieving and maintaining emotional and psychological balance. It is called Collar Bone breathing (CB2) and should be done each morning when you wake and at night. You may find it helps to set you up for the day and at night helps you sleep better:

Place 2 fingers of one hand on your collarbone (see pg 43) – keep the thumb clear & tap the gamut spot continuously whilst doing the following breathing pattern (seee Fig. 1):

      Take a full breath in – hold

      Let half breath out – hold

      Let all breath out – hold

      Take half breath in – hold

      Breathe out normally

Slide fingers across to other collarbone and repeat tapping and breathing (see Fig 2).

Fold fingers under, so knuckles touch collarbone (see pg 44) – keep thumb clear and repeat breathing sequence whilst tapping gamut spot. Slide to other collarbone and repeat (see Figs. 3 and 4).

fingers/fingers—knuckles/knuckles

Repeat other hand.

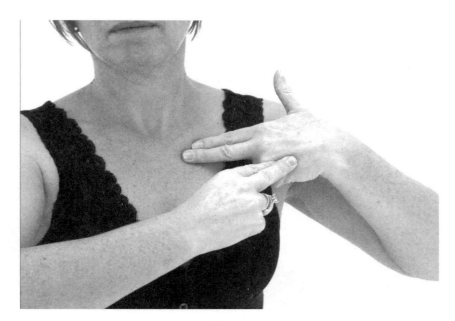

Fig. 1

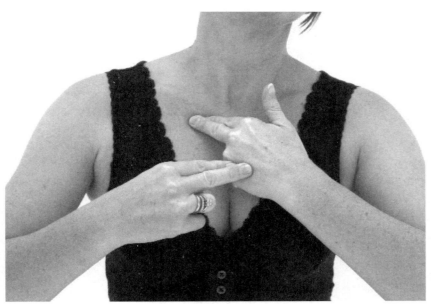

Fig. 2

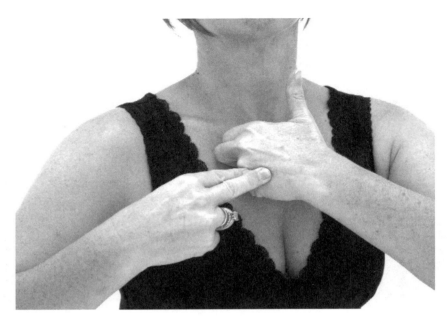

Fig. 3

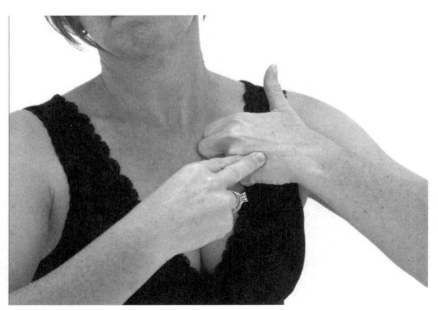

Fig. 4

Once you know you are committed and positive about losing weight, there is another thing you need to do: You need to **TELL PEOPLE** you are changing your behaviour otherwise they will encourage you to do as you did before. They know that you have "dieted" before so make sure you tell them you are **changing the way you eat, not that you are on a diet. A good example would be to say "I am looking after myself better" rather than "I am on a diet"**

You can also tell them about your new life goals – more about this later in the book. You will notice people start to treat you completely differently, at first with confusion, or maybe even disbelief, then with respect and admiration as they recognise how positive your changes are. You will find that other people start to ask you how you are doing it! You will inspire other people to do the same as you. How good does that feel knowing that through **your** actions other people can feel as good as you! Get them on side and you will save yourself potential aggravation and gain help and support.

CARELESS TALK

We all have it, that ceaseless chatter that goes on in our heads. It's totally normal. It's called your "inner voice" or "running commentary". It is NOT someone else inside your head telling you how to think or behave – it is a collection of all your experiences and influences that are fed back to you vocally in your mind. The most amazing thing I discovered throughout the last few years whilst I have been developing this programme is that people are often surprised to find out you can actually control your inner voice, and change it at will. Try this simple test:

- using your inner voice count to ten

- now count to ten but miss out the number four

- now give yourself a sexy French accent as you count – still missing out number four

So you see! You can get it to say whatever you want. If you don't put any effort into controlling how you talk to yourself, you will just feedback what others have told you, even if its not true or is unhelpful: For example if as a child you were told you were stupid on your first day of school, you would have been in "peak state" due to the nerves and anticipation so this would have locked in to your subconscious, after all we assume our teachers know what they are talking about, so if they say you are stupid they must be right (or not!). It doesn't take many repetitions of people saying you are stupid before your brain accepts this and continually feeds this back to you via your inner voice UNLESS *you* control what you accept as true. In later life if you want to try something new and challenging, you may not because you think you are "too stupid" to be able to do it, you may not apply for that promotion because you think you do not deserve it. It may be your friends or even your spouse that talk to you either intentionally or deliberately, in a way that tells you they have a low opinion of you. You may have allowed them to do this if you thought it's all you deserved. If this is the case it is probably because they heard you talking about yourself in a negative way, so this set the tone for them to do the same. You inadvertently gave them permission – more than that you showed them how to do it. How you talk to yourself to a very large extent determines how other people talk to you. As we have discussed if you are psychologically reversed you are more likely to feel negative about yourself and run even more negative chatter. Each time you hear yourself doing it, tap the side of your hand 15–20 times. Then go inside your head and tell your negative voice to SOD OFF.

Your brain responds to your inner voice, if it tells you that you should feel bad because you are fat, then you do, after all you don't want to call yourself a liar!

> The language you use when you talk to yourself is what determines how you feel and react.

Your brain will only respond to positive commands. If you type into your computers search engine "don't find a file named cats" then it brings up a list of sites about cats, trust me I just tried it on Google to make sure. In the same way if you say to your brain "don't eat too much" guess what message actually reaches your brain? All it hears is "eat too much". Say to a child "don't spill your drink" and what usually happens? They spill their drink. If you say "put your drink somewhere safe" they are more likely to put their drink in the centre of the table where it is less likely to get knocked off. What you can learn from this now, is to think in positive terms, not what you *should not* do, but what you *must* do instead. If you want to eat smaller portions rather than saying "don't eat too much" try saying "eat a bit less" and you will learn to eat less.

Your brain does not compute the meaning of "DON'T" it just sees "DO"

It's important to think in terms of what you need to *DO* and not what you need to stop doing.

YOUR LANGUAGE – TALK THE TALK

In the earlier chapter we discussed telling people around you what and how you are changing. Telling other people is important but not as important as what you tell yourself. How you control your internal chatter is the biggest single influence on your behaviour. Here are the two sentences again:

"I am on a diet"

"I am looking after myself better"

If you just look at the grammar of the sentences above you can see a subtle but critical difference: If you say you are "on" something then it is automatically assumed (by your brain and everyone else) that you can come "off" it at any time. e.g. when you are "on" a course of antibiotics, you know when you feel better you will come "off" them. If you are "on" a diet your brain is conditioned to think at some point you can and will come "off" it. However if you say you *are* something then that represents who you are in a *permanent* sense. Look at the following two sentences and see the difference in their underlying meaning ....

- I am fat

- I eat too much

Which way of speaking do you think is going to help you to change? If you tell yourself you are fat, then tell yourself to eat something healthy, you are giving your brain mixed messages. Your brain will want to defend the statement "I am fat" after all you don't want to be a liar, so it will influence your behaviour to support the fact you are fat. If you continue to use this language, losing weight for you is going to be like swimming against the tide. If on the other hand you change your language to "I ate too much" and "I feel better now I eat less" then it will be like letting the waves carry you forward toward your goal.

What is the difference between these two statements?

• "I am going to start eating healthily"

• "I am a healthy eater"

The first is something you plan to do, and the second is WHO YOU ARE. There is a big difference between the two, as you read this now, who are you? Are you someone who is *going to start* behaving like a healthy person sometime soon, or are you someone that even whilst reading this book, you are becoming a healthy person with new behaviours? It is not important if you have not started those new behaviours yet in the physical sense, your brain has undergone some re-wiring since you started working through this book and *you know you are different right now.* You are changing your mind.

If you have been "doing" not reading this book then you are re-wiring your mind. You already ARE healthier.

Healthy thinkers make healthy eaters, healthy eaters have healthy bodies,

Healthy bodies look good, looking good makes you feel good.

Everything you do in life is based on a desire to feel good.

I have never met a person who constantly talked in a negative way, thought about unhealthy foods all the time and managed to lose weight. What if you knew it's how you feel about food when you are *not* eating that influences what and how much you eat, more than what you think when you are actually eating. People who shovel in food without even tasting it usually eat far more than they need. People who eat slowly, thinking about what they are eating, eat less.

Questions are a powerful weapon

Positive statements and affirmations can be very useful in self development, as long as they are carefully structured and reflect *exactly* what you need to hear. What need to come BEFORE positive statements however, are QUESTIONS. Asking the right question is a vital part of developing a strategy or plan of action that will take you where you want to go.

My guess is that your self esteem has been quite low if you are not happy with how you look. Now you have begun some of the exercises, in particular the TFT and the visualization exercises and you can see "you" in the future, and how you are changing. However you need to be aware of the pitfalls that bring about low self esteem, so you can avoid them in the future and continue to achieve your personal goals. Any journey can have unexpected traffic jams, hold ups or diversions. When you are in such a situation you can either sit there and wait, getting frustrated or angry and "blaming" things around you, or you can ask yourself "how can I go around this obstacle and find a better way to get to where I want".

Making statements with your inner voice keeps you exactly where you are. If you are telling yourself something negative (or others are telling you and you believe and accept what they say), then your brain acts to support this "fact". This means if the statement is "I am fat" your subconscious will guide you towards behaviours to support this view. Conversely if you are saying to yourself "I am healthy" you get a quite different set of behaviours. In this way, positive statements or affirmations can stimulate the "right" behaviour. It is almost a robotic response to a command, **what your brain hears – it does.**

If you find yourself making negative statements, you can ask a positive question to turn it around and get a positive statement, and therefore a positive response in your behavior: for example:

"I am fat" becomes "I am fat, so how can I become slim....."

This is a great start and may help you, depending on one crucial factor, that is whether or not you LIKE the answer you get back! If the answer you get back is "I can go on a diet" and you immediately access memory patterns for diets that have caused you pain, your subconscious says "No thanks very much" and nothing changes in your behaviour because the thought of the diet causes you pain. As we have already discussed, your subconscious will automatically avoid behaviours that it knows will cause you pain, even if you have a "conscious" reason for wanting to do it. You may be able to "over-ride" this reluctance for a very short time, but it will not become part of your automatic behaviours and won't lead to long term change. The good news is that there is an easy way to get around this, which is to add three words to the end of every question so it becomes: "How can I become slim **AND ENJOY IT"**, now your brain searches its files for a way you can lose weight and *not experience pain.* A much better option! The answers may come straight away, or they may come over time as you increase your experiences and try out and learn new behaviours. Keep asking the right questions and the right answers will come. For example if you ask "how can I lose weight and enjoy it?" you may get an answer that's something like this "I can eat less *most* of the time and its OK to have unhealthy foods sometimes" this is much more appealing and more likely to bring about sustainable change.

In addition to what you say, *HOW* you say it is very important. In any given conversation (either with yourself internally or someone else externally) the words you use represent less than 10% of the information you give or receive. More important is HOW you speak, the intonation or the tone of your voice, the different emphasis or accent you put on different words, and most influential of all non verbal signals such as posture, body language, blushing, eye movements etc. Saying the right thing and "talking the talk" is important but HOW you communicate "words" is a vital part of that process. Have you ever said something to a friend or relative that they have "taken the wrong way", when the message you thought you delivered was totally different from the message they received?

This is called a METAMESSAGE. That is what actually gets

received in spite of what was said. Let me give you an example of a metamessage: I had been having some problems with my back and my chiropractor decided I needed some new molded insoles for my trainers as mine were ten years old, and recommended an excellent podiatrist. He gave me the number and when I got home I called it – I asked if I could make an appointment to see Mr Johnstone and got this response from the receptionist, given in a very austere tone of voice:

> "Mr. Johnstone no longer works here, in fact we have absolutely NO IDEA where he is, we have no contact with him and no forwarding address, his wife still works here and offers exactly the same treatment....... I can make an appointment with Mrs Johnstone..."

Hows that for a metamessage! That's what you might call "Too much information!" or as my daughter would say "Over-share!" even though she didn't tell me they have had an acrimonious divorce or separation and gone their separate ways, I found all that out not in the actual words she used, but by the tone and style with which they were delivered. I didn't make an appointment.

I can think of numerous times as a child when myself my brother and sister were told to "apologise to each other RIGHT NOW" and we crossed our arms, fired off glares at each other and in the most hostile tone we could summon uttered the painful word "sorry" to which we often got from my mother "Now say it again as if you mean it!" Even at that young age we instinctively knew the importance of the metamessage.

Repeat the following phrase in your head using your inner voice, keep the tone boring and plain and your body language still and face expressionless:

> "I am power – I can achieve anything"

How do you feel, did you believe what you said? What was your metamessage?

Now repeat this phrase as if you were an Olympic athlete who has just won a Gold Medal, who is physically jumping about, eyes wide open and fully animated – get into state:

"*I* **am** *power –* *I* **can** *achieve* **anything**"

How did you feel? Did you believe what you said – what was your metamessage?

Everyday we have conversations with people and we get the impression they don't mean what they say. When was the last time someone spoke to you and their metamessage was completely different from the words alone?

From now on you can control your own metamessages – by developing a radar that bleeps every time you say something to yourself in a way you don't actually mean – when you catch yourself doing "negative chatter" tap the side of your hand 15-20 times, then change your state in a way that makes you feel good, for example think of your happiest moment, or think of a time when you laughed till you couldn't stop, or a time when you achieved something you were proud of, and repeat a positive phrase in this style – say it like you mean it. The impact this has on the metamessage is massive and because you are "in state" your brain receptors are more active, your brain juice is flowing and the intended positive message goes in you mind.

The word used to describe when speech matches actions is CONGRUENT. If someone is telling you about a product they want you to buy, even if they have their sales patter memorised, but they don't believe in the value of their product you can just sense it. This is because your brain is picking up lots of little signals you are not even aware of such as eye movements and even the smallest changes in body language. This person is INCONGRUENT, that is their actions contradict the message they are trying to get across. You simply don't believe them, or more specifically you don't believe *they* believe what they say.

You often see these two qualities in politicians, we instinctively trust the ones who are congruent and they are the ones who get our vote. The last time you voted, either national, council or even for a local school governor was your decision based on their policies alone? Did you go on the internet and read the manifestos carefully before you made your decision? Or if it was a local committee did you talk personally to each candidate about what they would do? Or did you vote for who you instinctively felt was honest and had integrity and meant what they said - even if you didn't agree with all of their policies or even some of their actions. Did you believe that *they* believed they were genuinely doing the right thing? If this was your view of them, irrespective of policy then they were CONGRUENT, in your mind they *meant what they said.*

On the other hand why did you not vote for the other candidates? Did you not believe they would be able to carry out what they said? Was there something about them that you just didn't want to put your trust in? Did you think they were only saying certain things to win votes and they didn't really believe it themselves? Was there something that was "just not right" about them? If so they were INCONGRUENT.

When you are talking to yourself, especially if you are re-wiring your brain, you must BE CONGRUENT, you have to mean what you say 100% and more. You must change your voice, be strong and positive, you must physically stand tall or sit up straight, mind body and soul must be united in delivering the message for it to have the desired effect.

Not only can you change the words you use in your internal chatter, but you can give yourself any accent tone or volume you want. Most people think that their internal chatter is just "there", it has its voice, it sounds a certain way and cannot be changed. The good news is IT CAN BE CHANGED and YOU can change it, and doing so completely changes the effect it has on you and your thoughts and actions. Changing the effect negative chatter has on how you behave is easy if you change the way you say it.

In the box below write down a negative commentary that you

regularly run, you will almost certainly have a list of unflattering comments that you believe to be true that you say about yourself:

Your negative commentary

_____

_____

_____

Now read it and say it to yourself exactly as you normally do, copy your tone of voice and actually hear yourself saying the words.

How does that make you feel? What is the metamessage, what are you hearing? Exactly with what is being said? what is under the surface of the language? the deeper meaning in addition to the words you have used? How much authority and control over you does this voice have, how does it make you feel? On a scale of 1–10 how much negative influence does this statement said in this way, have over your behaviour, thoughts and feelings? Circle the correct number:

No Influence   **Maximum Influence**
(negative)   **(positive)**

1	2	3	4	5	6	7	8	9	10

Tap the side of your hand 15–20 times: Now change your inner voice to something you find ridiculous and give it an image, I will give you an example but if you can think of a character or style more ridiculous use that instead: become a speaking mouse, with a tiny twittery squeaky voice, who is trying to stand on its back 2 legs and keeps falling over and getting back up, the mouse is very small and grey and looks very weak

---

physically. Now add some humour, think of something very slapstick that would make you laugh. Get the image and the voice clearly in your mind – practice counting to 10 in this squeaky insignificant voice to make sure it sounds ridiculous enough. * *Now re-read the negative chatter in this voice and this style.*

It sounds really stupid doesn't it? Hearing it like this how much or how little authority does this voice have? How much do you believe what it says is true?

On a scale of 1-10 how much influence does this voice have over your behaviour, thoughts and feelings? Circle the correct number:

1	2	3	4	5	6	7	8	9	10

Now make this mouse even smaller, so small you can barely even see it, make the image black and white, make the silly squeaky voice even more ridiculous and repeat the phrase again. On a scale of 1-10 how much influence does this voice have over your behaviour thoughts and feelings now? Circle the correct number:

1	2	3	4	5	6	7	8	9	10

If the number you circle is above 1, keep repeating the exercise making the mouse and voice smaller and smaller and less and less significant until it is nothing except ridiculous and insignificant, with no authority or control or influence over you whatsoever. In other words keep doing whatever you need to do to change it, until all authority in it has gone and you instinctively "know" whatever it says has no meaning. Make it truly pathetic.

Once you have deleted the negative chatter and feelings you must replace them with something positive: you can make a statement more powerful using visionary and imaginary skills:

Fill in the box below what you would most like to achieve in your life (weight loss or otherwise). Do it in positive current or future tense, e.g.;

"I will lose three dress sizes, I will do this, and I am going to find a way to enjoy the process and make it fun".

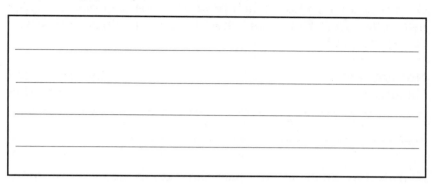

Now read it back in the style you normally use when talking to yourself, get the tone of your usual negative inner voice exactly right On a scale of 1 – 10 how much do you believe in your ability to achieve that goal?

Negative   **Positive**

1	2	3	4	5	6	7	8	9	10

Now change your state. If you saw the cartoon Aladdin when Robin Williams played the voice of the genie, it was so loud and booming that Aladdin was literally blown off his feet when he spoke! Your brain is great at creating cartoon type images, so use any techniques you need to make it totally believable, as you create in your mind a genie with real powers. You may need your genie to be beautiful, and majestic, dressed in bright glittering colours, standing tall and strong, so you *know* that your internal genie can make *anything* happen just by uttering the words, **"your wish is my command"**. Once you have got into state – remember "pretend" is fine as long as you pretend intensely, so for the next few moments you ARE that genie –

now go back and re-read the phrase in the style of the genie of the lamp.

How does that make you feel, have you changed your "brain juice"?

On a scale of 1–10 how much positive influence does this voice have over your behaviour, thoughts and feelings? Circle the correct number:

Not bothered   **Fully committed**
Negative   **Positive**

1	2	3	4	5	6	7	8	9	10

If it is less than 10, go back and do it again with more commitment, more energy and more enthusiasm and get more ASSOCIATED into the process. Believe it, even if you have to pretend you believe it, it will work. Keep going until you have achieved a perfect 10.

Be careful what you say to yourself – you may be listening

Remember that no-one else ever hears how you talk to yourself, so using images and borrowing other people's voices is absolutely fine. If it makes you smile and you have fun even better – why not feel good for no apparent reason?

Using TFT to eliminate low self esteem
I use this technique with almost all of my clients, whether they want to lose weight or not. In my experience most people who suffer negative emotions, from anxiety or depression, to phobias, have some reduced levels of self esteem that holds them back and stops them achieving their goals and desires. Eliminating low self esteem is one of the most empowering things you can do and it's possible with TFT.

Exercise
Stand in front of a mirror and think about how you feel about

yourself. Give yourself a SUD rating of 1–10 with 10 being full of negativity and bad feelings about yourself and 1 being no bad feelings. In other words the higher the number the lower the self esteem or the worse you feel about yourself. Using the procedure and points shown on page .... Tap the following sequence whilst looking in the mirror and focusing on the negative feelings you feel about yourself:

- Side hand (karate spot)
- Under eye
- Under arm
- Collar bone
- Under nose
- Under lip
- Collar bone
- Middle finger
- 9g
- Repeat sequence.

Take a new SUD. If the negative feelings are less repeat the treatment exactly until it is eliminated. If the SUD is still the same, tap the side of the hand, then rub the sore spot just under the left collar bone, then tap under the nose and start the process again from the beginning.

Positive Imagery Exercise
This simple exercise is a great way of teaching yourself to feel good about yourself – for no reason whatsoever!

Raise the right arm up and to the right of you so you are looking up at your hand.... look into your palm and create a compelling image of what you want to be like, assuming that nothing can fail and you will be successful.

Then double the intensity of the picture in your right hand and brighten it. Then double it again and again...when it looks amazing, and only then, take a deep breath in and as you exhale, physically move your arm and pull the image into you, place your hand on your chest and absorb the image into your heart, then as you breathe in, intensify the image, as you exhale drive the picture and the feeling through your body into every cell, muscle, nerve fibre and tissue until you are saturated with the good feeling. Then repeat with another good image. Layer in good feeling after good feeling.

Do this as often as you like - after all who can ever have enough good feelings? **Next time someone says "keep your chin up" they may be talking more sense than they realise, changing your physical state is a vital part of changing your mental state.**

Now think about your future in the positive state, think about your job, your relationships, your personal goals: staying in positive state how do you feel about your future? Remember how you feel is a choice – your choice.

Practice feeling good – for no reason whatsoever!

THINKING DIFFERENTLY

Are you a glass half full or a glass half empty thinker? We often hear the term "Positive Thinker" and it is certainly useful to see the best in everything as it gives us more options: at the same time if things are bleak (and bad things happen even to positive people!) we need to be able to deal with it in the most positive way possible. The term used for 'thinking differently' or 'seeing things from a different perspective' is REFRAMING, which means taking the situation, looking at it carefully and finding something positive you can take from it either now, or as a reference point for the future. People who do not have the skills to reframe generally either bury their head in the sand and pretend its not happening, or become so negative they can only see doom and gloom when bad things happen.

An example of someone who has a good sense of reframing is Billy Connolly when he says "There's no such thing as bad weather – just times when you are wearing the wrong clothes!" The comedians that make us laugh the most are often the ones that take everyday situations and reframe them to give them a humorous perspective that we can all relate to.

What experiences have you had in the past that you need to reframe in order to put them behind you and move on? This programme is designed to focus on weight loss but you are have already learning many skills that are going to help you in all aspects of your life. You may have negative associations based on previous diets you have tried, you have memory patterns that had sabotaged your subsequent attempts at changing your shape, but all those experiences can be reframed in an instant: you can choose to change.

We learn from our mistakes and those who accept this knowledge gracefully and see it as an asset move forward, wiser for the experience. Those who cannot reframe and constantly moan about how "unlucky" they are stay where they are in a negative state and effectively lock "good luck" out.

Think of something negative that has happened to you that has been festering in your mind and holding you back. Now reframe, find something (however small) that has happened or could happen as a result and focus on it. How can you use that reframe to move you forward, has that piece of knowledge or experience been lying dormant? What can you do today to start benefiting from it? The past is behind you. You alone choose what to take with you into the future.

Everything you have learned so far in this book is making you stronger and you are changing, probably more than you realise. Some of the messages will have gone into your subconscious mind and you begin to change, doubt and question some of your previous thinking.

Now you are ready for the next level, for which you need two more things: first you need a definite goal and second you need a strategy. The first part we will deal with now, the second includes the nutrition and eating plan *you* are going to create in the next chapters, based on foods you enjoy and living a life you want to live, in a body you want to live in.

SET GOALS YOU WILL BE
COMPELLED TO ACHIEVE

This chapter is dynamite. When you have completed this section you will be a million miles away from where you were before you started working through this book. More than any other this is a chapter you DO as opposed to a chapter you just read, so come on and DO IT!!

Many years experience working for national diet & fitness clubs, in my own health clubs and with hundreds of individual clients, has taught me a lot about goal setting: I have watched and studied clients and identified a clear pattern and set of behaviours and beliefs that separates those who achieve their goals from those who don't. I can share those differences with you now, so that YOU are someone who achieves their goals.

It is important to make sure that the goal you set fits in with your Beliefs and your Values. In this section of the book you will work out what is important to you, what you believe you CAN do, not what you believe you cannot do. As a result you will be able to set goals that make you feel not just quite good, but absolutely fantastic! Forget any previous goals you may have had, they probably weren't inspirational enough or important enough to you anyway, that's why you haven't achieved them yet. The goals you set for yourself from now on will absolutely change your life – so get excited!

Are You Unbelievable?
Beliefs are "things" you believe, or *know* beyond doubt to be true. Your belief structure dictates how you think and act and forms the basis for your habitual behaviours. You believe this book is helping you, you are continuing with it because you want to change. That's a good decision, based on a belief. Many times we make bad decisions based on beliefs. Beliefs are not always positive: consider the many people in Waco in

America who took their own lives; they didn't do this on a whim, they did it because they believed in their cause and that it was the right thing to do. Most of us cannot comprehend that strength of belief or conviction, to be so sure of something that you would not only kill yourself but in some cases take the lives of your own children as well. That's a pretty powerful belief.

Conversely there have been people in history who have had such strong beliefs that their behaviour and the way they lived their lives changed the way you and I live our lives today for good. Amongst the people we have to thank are:

- Christopher Columbus for believing the World was round not flat.

- Thomas Edison for believing that light could be transmitted through a bulb.

- Martin Luther King for believing the colour of your skin doesn't make you less of a person.

- Christian Barnard for believing it was possible to take a heart or other organ out of one body and transplant it successfully into another.

- Emmeline Pankhurst for believing women should have the same rights to vote as men.

Without people questioning traditionally held beliefs we might still believe the world was flat, or that man could never travel to the moon, or that it isn't possible to run a mile in less than four minutes! We have Roger Bannister to thank for that one: interestingly as soon as he shattered that belief and proved it could be done, within months other athletes were achieving the same seemingly "impossible" task. Now when elite athletes train for this distance they *expect* to be sub four minutes. When you consider beliefs in these terms you begin to see how important it is when goal setting, to have a well formed belief system that works on the basis of what you *can do*.

BELIEFS ARE POWER

they can be positive or negative in equal strength

Beliefs are formed during childhood. When we are children we believe we are capable of absolutely *anything* until the grown ups teach us otherwise and start putting limits on our behaviour.

- don't touch the oven

- don't run across the road

- don't go near the water's edge

We are taught not to do so many things that it becomes almost second nature to think about everything in negative terms: even though these are very "good" instructions that teach us how to be safe, taking this concept into every aspect of our life i.e. focusing on what we "can't do" can lead to us developing a string of negative beliefs.

When you fail at something more than once, it can lead to a belief that you will never be able to do it. Once you believe you cannot do something you stop trying, in-fact you often subconsciously avoid anything connected with this "thing" to protect yourself against the pain of failure: in this way your negative or limiting belief becomes a self fulfilling prophecy. You think you can't, therefore you can't.

The nature of limiting beliefs is that once you have them you "honour" them in a way that stops you progressing or achieving what you truly desire.

What don't you believe you can achieve?

Complete the first part of the following statement – be honest:

I would like to _____

but I don't believe I can because...

The *because* part of the sentence, which automatically comes next in your internal chatter, is how you justify this limiting belief. These comments are based on past experiences or observations that you have accepted as the only outcome of you trying to achieve your goal. In coaching many people approach this part of the sentence first, and that can work well: however it can be quicker and more beneficial to address the limiting belief head on and not bother with the "*because*" part. In my experience the word "because" often precedes a torrent of verbal bullshit, either from internal chatter or words someone actually verbalises when telling me why they can't achieve something. Of course there are times when it is a perfectly acceptable phrase. For example:

Q. why can't you fly?

A. because I don't have wings.

BUT.... often it is used to justify your failure to achieve a certain task. How many times have you heard yourself say "I can't do that because........" and then proceed to give excuses/reasons why not, many if not all of which could be overcome if your life depended on it.

Internal chatter contributes to the beliefs we form about what we can or cannot achieve: when it comes to vocabulary, whether internal or external, it's much more helpful to ask "How can I?" rather than "Why can't I?" Even better ask yourself "How can I...... and enjoy it!" When you ask your brain a question it will respond with an answer. Often we don't ask the question because we don't want to hear the answer, as it might tell us to do something we don't want to do.

Asking yourself the right questions is important if you want to grow and develop as a person. If you just make statements, such as "I am fat" that won't help you achieve anything except low self esteem, but if you turn it into a question such as "How can I lose fat and still enjoy myself?" you get a completely different response. Next time you look in the mirror and say "I am fat" have your internal voice say something like "Yes I know that, now *what can I do about it that involves having fun*!"

If you hear yourself using the word "because", have your internal alarm bells go off and think carefully about exactly what you are saying.

The following exercise is called "Swish", it works quickly and effectively to enable you to see and believe, you can achieve whatever you want. As with all exercises you will need to fully focus using your three filters:

The Swish

1.   Identify a limiting belief you currently hold. It must be something you believe you cannot do or achieve, not something you think you may be able to do or could do if or when...... you need to genuinely believe you are not capable of doing this behaviour AT ALL. Inside your minds eye make a picture of yourself not being able to do the behaviour you have identified – the thing you believe you cannot do: **Be associated (view through your own eyes).** Now reduce this image to the bottom left of your vision much like you would minimise an image on a computer screen

2.   Make a picture of how you would like to be. Make it a compelling desirable picture that shows you behaving in ways that guarantee success. Make it bigger, bolder and better: see how happy you are having achieved all the changes you want. Look at yourself through the eyes of an observer, **be disassociated as if you are watching a movie of you.** Settle on the most compelling aspect and freeze frame it into a picture, something that when you see it fills you with pride and create a desire to be just like that image.

3.   Reduce the 2nd desirable picture and bring up the 1st picture, but keep the desirable picture in its reduced form in the bottom left corner. Be aware its there.

As you focus on the negative picture have the desirable picture *suddenly explode into your vision* literally knocking out the negative picture and be overwhelmed by how much you desire it, then blank both pictures out completely and imagine a plain white screen.

4.   Repeat the "swishing" technique at least 5 times.

5.   When you automatically "swish" to the desirable picture everytime you try in vain to see the picture you want to change, you have succeeded.

If you believe you want to, need to and importantly are *going to* change your shape, then you need to change some behaviours and that involves changing a few long held beliefs: first you need to believe you will succeed, I have shown you how to do that in a variety of ways, and there's still more to come.........to be 100% successful you need to align your behaviours with your beliefs, then it will not only be easy to change, you will be compelled to change. If you believe that behaving in a certain way will move you towards your goal and towards the PLEASURE end of the pleasure / pain scale, then changing the belief will become automatic. If you doubt the benefit of a new behaviour and you don't believe it will profit you, then you are unlikely to do it often enough for it to become automatic, therefore it will not work and you will fulfil your doubt and justify your failure to change – it wasn't *you* it was the diet! The amount of times I have heard people say "dieting didn't work for me" when in reality any diet that reduces what you eat causes you to lose weight – although whether its healthy or not is a different matter. One of the basic laws of physics relates to energy balance and no human being opposes this law:

If you eat less calories than you burn you lose weight.

This is one belief it's worth holding onto. By accepting this you are accepting responsibility for your size and shape and acknowledging that if you are fat it is because you ate too much and were not active enough. It doesn't make you a bad person; it just means you got fat.

Your body is a way of showing you and everyone else how you live your life. What does your body say about you? How is that different from what you would like it to say about you? You have a choice whether to stay doing the same behaviours you did and staying the same size and shape, or changing your behaviours and changing your size and shape. Life is a choice.

If you have the complete WLIM system listen to CD2 'Treasure Chest' now. See audio information sheet at the back of the book for more information.

TAKE BACK YOUR POWER

To be successful you first have to believe that what you change will guarantee you achieve your goal and second that you will enjoy the changes so they will become habitual. This means you will automatically do the new behaviours without thinking. Using Weight Loss In Mind techniques will make this process much easier and make will power redundant, CHANGE is the only power you need.

HOW VALUABLE ARE YOUR VALUES?

Values are inextricably linked with **Beliefs** and also underpin the way we think and act. They are not morals or principles they are just instinctive feelings or a "sense" of something that you know feels "right" for you. They may be described as qualities or characteristics but they are not tangible, they are not material things, so if someone says they value their car for example, you would need to ask what feelings they get from the car. If it is a sports car they may say speed, or danger, if it is a Bentley they may say comfort or security: People with different values buy different cars, different houses, have different jobs and different friends. Of course that is not to say that all your friends have the same values as you, but almost certainly they will have *some* of the same values as you. You will have things in common you like, or hobbies you share, these are all based on your values. People are naturally drawn to other people who are like them, its human nature. Your first conversation with someone new is based around you each finding what about the other person is "like" you. The more you have in common, the better the rapport you develop and the more the chance you will develop a longer term relationship. When you communicate with another person for the first time and discover they have the same values as you, you have a connection with that person.

In Life Coaching there are several techniques to elicit values, but I have always found this one to be the most enjoyable, least restrictive and the most effective because it requires you to let go of any boundaries and let your imagination loose:

Exercise

Have a pen and paper ready. Sit quietly for a few minutes and daydream about your perfect day, a day of absolute bliss where you experience everything that is important to you. Delete the normal restrictions of finance ability or location. This means if you want breakfast on the moon and the afternoon in the Bahamas you can -anything is possible. Imagine precisely what your perfect day would be like. Start when you wake up – where are you? who are you with? what is your first thought? Take yourself through the day in your mind including everything and anything that would have to happen to make it a perfect day. Go right through the morning, afternoon and evening until you climb into bed at the end of the day. Include everything that you would do or experience in your perfect day. When you have finished do a mental check back, is there anything else that could have happened that would have made it even better? Once you have a clear idea write it all down, from waking till sleeping, every bit. Now read it back, look at each event and think about the feeling or sense that event gave you: for example if you were skydiving what *feeling* did that give you? Perhaps it might be adventure or danger, if you love either of these and it without these experiences it wouldn't be your perfect day then adventure and or danger are values for you. Or perhaps if you were with someone you can show love to and who loves you what feeling did that give you? Love itself is not a value, its too broad a word, its what is known as a "chunk" word which means you can break it down into smaller chunks and get other things from it, for example giving love may mean a feeling or sense of caring or nurturing, or feeling loved may mean feeling valued or appreciated. Did you do something that made you proud? Did you achieve something? Or did you just find contentment doing very simple things? Did you have a sense of peace? Or did you have a sense of excitement or challenge? These are suggestions but there are many more feelings you can have. It is common to have two apparently opposite feelings; one event may have given you excitement while another later in the same day may have given you peace and both are important to you. You will probably end up with between six and eight feelings that you would just HAVE to have it were to be the absolute PERFECT day.

Now think about all the people you love and admire. The ones you know and maybe some you see from afar and have never met. What characteristics or qualities MUST they have for you to admire them? What values must people have in their character that you aspire to or, already have and hold dear?

Use the table below to help you, on the left hand side write what you did/saw/heard and in the right hand column write the feeling or sense this activity or experience gave you. Then add the characteristics you value in yourself and others.

Here are some examples to help you get the idea. It's important to write what you genuinely feel, not what you "think" you should value.

Event/Activity/Experience	"Sense" or "Feeling" = Value
Walking down a beautiful beach	Sense of Peace
Surfing a huge wave	Sense of Adventure
Being with my family	Giving love/caring nurturing or Receiving love/ being appreciated or valued, or feeling safe or secure
Writing a song	Sense of Achievement
Observing nature	Sense of appreciating Creation
Characteristics	
Honesty	Trust
Loving	Ambition
Sense of fun and humour	Generous

Recognise that you may have conflicting values, you may for example love sky diving and adventure, but also love just looking at the stars at night and enjoying a sense of peace. They don't have to make sense or even compliment each other, there may or may not be lots of variety between your values, just go with your instinct.

Event/Activity/Experience	"Sense" or "Feeling" = Value
Characteristics	

When you have completed the table do a mental check to see if there's anything you have missed out, make any alterations and then transfer your list of values to the table below, in no particular order of importance. If you have more than eight, pick the eight most important. Some people only have four or five so just go with your instinct.

Core Values

These are your **CORE VALUES**, feelings or qualities you instinctively hold dear. If you live your life in accordance with your values you can live in peace. If you live and act in opposition to your values you will be under stress and find it difficult to relax. For example if one of your values is to feel healthy, then being fat and or unhealthy will cause you distress. If you do not value health but beauty in the human form or in any other form is of value to you, then again being fat will cause you distress if you believe it compromises beauty. If you value honesty and integrity yet work for a company or boss who asks you to lie to get clients, that will cause you stress.

At different times in your life different values will have priority, especially if they slightly contrast each other: for example some of my values are loving and giving which I fulfil when I am with my family, but I also value personal development and achievement, contributing and making a difference to others, which means I sometimes need to spend time away from my family. At different times you need different things, for example work may satisfy one value, whereas home life or relationships another. This is powerful stuff so take your time as you do this exercise well.

When you have completed the list and have your "core values" then ask yourself honestly, "Am I honouring this value in my life now?" by which I mean are you doing something regularly that gives you this feeling or sense. Put a tick or a cross in the column on the right. For those that have a cross beside them, you need to think about what behaviour or activity you will do in your life to make sure you honour this value at least some of the time.

When you design your strategy i.e. which behaviours you are going to change to achieve your weight loss, run each one past your list of values to make sure they are not in conflict: for example, if for exercise and calorie burning you have chosen to go for a power-walk every day for thirty minutes, and one of your core values is company/friendship and you dislike solitude, you should consider a more group based exercise, because with the best will in the world if you do not enjoy it you will not sustain it. Conversely if a sense of appreciating nature/creation is a value to you, then a walk by yourself every morning appreciating your surroundings in all seasons, watching the changing colours of the trees and plants etc. will bring you a deep sense of satisfaction. Of course you may (like me) value both these things therefore a mixture of group activity some days and solitary activity others is what you need.

Understanding what makes you happy is crucial for planning any behaviour change. This exercise also highlights what makes you unhappy and you may begin to see things that you do that cause you distress. Once you can identify these facets of your life you can stop them. For some people working out their values is a real light-bulb moment and it suddenly seems so clear why some things feel right and some don't. Understanding your values gives you a criteria for any decisions you need to make that will have a large impact on your life. If you are offered a new job, simply work out what that job will give you and see if it "fits" with your values. They are a blueprint for what makes you happy.

BELEIFS AND VALUES DETERMINE OUR GOALS

What is a goal?
If you say "My goal is to be rich" and you continue to go to work in the same shop/office/factory for years and rely on buying a

lottery ticket every week then you do not have a goal to be rich, you have a "wish" or a "hope". Unless you are proactive towards achieving it, it is not a goal it's a wish. If you "wish" you were slim but change nothing, then nothing changes.

It is unlikely that you will have one "global" goal that will bring you everything you want. If you think being slim is going to solve all your relationship problems, make you more successful at work, make you more intelligent etc. then you are mistaken. However, being slim may be a "personal" goal that brings you great satisfaction, a sense of achievement, raised self esteem and improved health. Within that category you can be 100% successful. You will need to have other goals as well if you desire wealth, increased intelligent etc. Putting goals into categories helps you to work out exactly what you want in life and allows you to accept success in some areas even if other areas still need work. If all your sense of achievement is dependant on one global goal then you are unlikely ever to feel you have accomplished.

Many clients come to me having been given a "target goal weight" by a slimming club, based solely on their height, with no consideration to body composition. Muscle is 2 $\frac{1}{2}$ times more dense than fat. This means you could have someone the size of Arnold Schwarzenegger weighing in at the same weight as someone the size of Robbie Coltrane. One of the personal trainers who used to work for me was 5ft 9 tall, weighed 11st 7lbs and had a figure anyone would kill for, as a well toned lean size 10-12. When clients would tell me they wanted to weigh ten stone I would ask Emma to come in and ask the client "would you rather weigh ten stone or look like this!"

Setting professional/work related goals is easier than setting personal goals such as weight loss or relationship goals, as you are more able to take the emotion out.

There is a mnuemonic that is often used in Life Coaching to help you set a goal:

SMART GOALS

S – SPECIFIC

M – MEASUREABLE

A – ACTION BASED

R – REALISTIC

T – TIME PHASED

SPECIFIC – this means instead of having a "vague" idea of what you want to achieve – you have a definite idea of exactly what dress size you want to be and a clear image in your mind of how you want to look.

Although scales can be a good guide, they must be used with common sense. When you look great and you are the dress size you have always wanted that must override anything the scales tell you. For this reason dress size is a better measure of success than scales, which can be notoriously inaccurate.

MEASUREABLE – You need to know how you are going to measure not just your final outcome, but more importantly your progress along the way. More important than how many inches you have lost, is measuring the success of your new patterns of behaviour, how successful have you been at exercising regularly? How successful have you been at eating less? If these things are happening results in terms of size and shape are guaranteed.

ACTION – that means what are you DOING to make it happen? What is your strategy? You already know you need to change your thinking, your internal chatter, how you visualise things and your behaviours or habits and in the following chapters you are going to develop a clear nutrition strategy, so you have everything you need to make the change.

TIME – this means being very clear not just about what and how, but *when* you want to achieve your desired results. When you know theres a deadline you become more focused. Without a deadline it's too easy to put things off.

Goals are a working document, that is they need to be flexible and aspects of them may need to change as you learn more about what works and what doesn't. A strategy that works for one person may not work for someone else: If your end goal is to lose three dress sizes, and your ACTION is to go to a club / gym / class three times per week, but you only ever mange two, instead of beating yourself up and thinking you have "failed" because you missed a gym visit you have several options:

•   The two times you do visit stay a bit longer so that the total time you spend at the gym in a week remains the same, you complete it in two visits instead of three

•   Find other times when you could be more active to compensate e.g. walk to work or to take children to school, have a game of badminton or play another sport with your partner so you don't have to take time out by yourself

•   Look carefully at your other commitments and see if there is anything that is less important to you that can be reduced or removed. If you *can't see* a way it doesn't mean there *isn't a way* it means there is a way but you haven't found it yet, so talk to someone who does achieve what you want to and open your eyes to different strategies you haven't considered before – maybe get up an hour earlier!

What "how can I" questions do you need to ask yourself now?

A few final points before you identify your exact weight/fat loss goal: it needs to be something positive, something you want to achieve rather than a negative, for example to be dress size 12 is a positive goal, i.e. to *be something*. An example of a negative goal would be "not to be fat". As discussed earlier it also needs to be realistic so when it comes to size ask yourself the following questions to make sure it is achievable:

• when was the last time you were this size?

• how long did you sustain this size for?

So if you are five feet ten inches and your goal is size 10, and as an adult you have never been a size 10, you need to reassess what is achievable and also whether you would look good as a size 10. Chances are you would look much better as a toned 12 or 14. Having said that BE AMBITIOUS, with this programme you really have got the POWER TO CHANGE not just your shape but your whole life. If I were to hit you over the head with a shovel now, so all your negative thoughts and beliefs in what you could not achieve were gone, if you opened your eyes with a blank screen for a mind and you suddenly found out you can genuinely achieve ANYTHING you want physically (apart from changing height!) what shape or size will you be?

Take a few moments to visualise people you know who are the size and shape (not weight) you would like to be. Once you have a clear idea of what that size looks like, picture yourself as that size, or you may have been this size and are able to look at a photograph – even better. The clearer the mental picture you have of what you are aiming for the better. Once you have got the image, you need to get the positive feelings you associate with being this size. It is actually the feeling that you want more than the size, you just need the size to give you the feeling so you acknowledge both. Now you know exactly what your physical and emotional goals are, the next step is to write them down.

Step 1.

My physical goal is_____

My emotional goal is to feel_____

Now you know what you need to do, its time to work out exactly when you are going to achieve it by.

The next step is to set a LONG TERM time frame, when MUST you achieve it by. Not "I hope to achieve it by..." or "I should achieve it by......." No wooliness or bullshit allowed, make a commitment now, when MUST and when WILL you absolutely achieve it by.

Step 2.

I MUST and WILL achieve my end goal by
    Physical   _____

    Emotional _____

The next step is to plan how you are going to measure your success, not just the end result, but along the way so you can see you are on course. This way if you drift off course you can pick it up, change your strategy to get back on track. For example it may be getting your partner/friend/relation to measure you each week. This part of the process must include some written record of your progress, either in journal form, a few paragraphs at least once per week, or a progress card that you have to show to at least one other person. Emotionally you need to monitor how good you feel about yourself. Making a scale from 1– 0 with 1 being the furthest away from your desired feeling you can imagine and 10 the full force of your desired feeling is a good way to monitor emotional progress. A simple piece of paper with lines of 1–10 on is all you need. If you have a better way of monitoring emotional progress that's great use that.

Step 3.

I am going to measure my progress by
Physical _____

Emotional _____

The next step is to redefine the behaviour goals you worked on earlier in the programme, you will have identified at least three core habitual behaviours you need to change by doing the earlier exercises (pages 35–36) but you can have as many as you need. You may decide to change all these behaviours in one go if you are an all or nothing personality, or if you are more methodical you may be more successful if you change one behaviour at a time.

Step 4.

I will achieve:
Behaviour change 1 by_____

Behaviour change 2 by_____

Behaviour change 3 by_____

Behaviour change 4 by_____

Behaviour change 5 by_____

Next you need to work out how often you are going to measure your progress other than the behaviour changes mentioned. I suggest weekly for the first 8 weeks, then fortnightly for the next 8 weeks and then monthly. This may not suit everyone and you may prefer to continue to check your progress weekly. Remember this doesn't have to mean being weighed every week slimming club style! If this works for you fine, but if it reminds you of slimming club diets that failed then you are linking the process with pain, STOP! PAIN IS NOT ALLOWED! In the next box put the exact dates of the first 12 stages/times when you are going to measure your progress. You will notice there is also space for a **comment**, this is where you write what you are doing that's working well, or make a note of something that didn't work.

As you are noting what is working for you i.e. giving you PLEASURE not PAIN make a "note to self" which maybe anything from an affirmation to an idea for something new to try, or something you have achieved or just how you feel: this information is important as each time you complete a Progress Check (PC) you can re-read it and remind yourself of what works *e.g:*

PC 1 = 14th January **comment** – *found out that if I have porridge or muesli I feel full up till lunchtime so didn't want a snack.* **note to self**: *I got in my jeans today for 1st time in years! Feel much better about myself, its really working!*

Step 5.

Progress check (PC) 1 (date) Comment Note to self	PC 5 Comment Note to self
PC 2 Comment Note to self	PC 6 Comment Note to self
PC 3 Comment Note to self	PC 7 Comment Note to self
PC 4 Comment Note to self	PC 8 Comment Note to self

PC 9	PC 11
Comment	Comment
Note to self	Note to self
PC 10	PC 12
Comment	Comment
Note to self	Note to self

- *PC. When you have completed these PCs **make a new table for the next 12 PCs.***

- *You will also need to come back to this table for the exercise at the end of this chapter.*

There are two checks that you need to do to finalise your preparation and clear the way for progress, and both of these checks involve other people.

The first is to look at your immediate circle i.e. family/friends and identify who will be affected by your new behaviours and in what way. If it is a negative effect, how can you alter it to be a positive effect? Bear in mind that if you have "dieted" before and failed, then those who love you will probably try and dissuade you from another attempt out of kindness because they don't want you to fail and get hurt: they don't yet know this programme is different from everything else you have tried. Alternatively, and this may not be easy to hear, they may also be fat, or unhappy with how they look or feel and as a result feel threatened at the prospect of you succeeding where they have failed. Out of a strong instinct for self preservation they may deter you from changing your behaviour, as if you succeed where they fail (or believe they will fail) it will make them feel inadequate. This may not be intentional on their part, but it's important you know that the person with the strongest desire will succeed, so *if their desire for you to fail is stronger than your desire to succeed, it will be so.* On the other hand if *your desire and importantly your BELIEF that you will succeed is stronger you will be.* Which will it be?

- Who close to you can benefit from you achieving your goal?

  _____

- How exactly will they benefit?

  _____

To wrap this section up and define your new sense of purpose, complete the following statements:

Physically I will *NO LONGER SETTLE FOR BEING*

_____

_____

Emotionally I will *NO LONGER SETTLE FOR FEELING*

_____

_____

Physically I will *ONLY SETTLE FOR BEING*

_____

_____

Emotionally I will *ONLY SETTLE FOR FEELING*

_____

_____

STRATEGY

Although I have designed a two week programme designed to give you a quick start and boost you physically and mentally, what you are learning is how to develop a permanent strategy that works for you. Strategies are a bit like a flight plan. A plane takes off from Heathrow heading for Los Angeles and it has a precise flight plan i.e. written details of exactly which path to take to ensure it gets to the correct destination. During the flight this plan is likely to change, as it passes through various different countries air space, it may be asked to bear north a few degrees, or south. There may be turbulence and the plane may have to climb higher to avoid strong winds, but each time there is a slight deviation, the route is recalculated to reach the same destination.

In the same way when I am using my sat nav in my car, if I take a wrong turn, it simply recalculates the route to take in my self imposed diversion and I continue. You may need to adapt your new strategy or "flight plan" as you meet unexpected diversions. Bear in mind some of these changes may actually be short cuts as you learn what works best for you!

On the basis you want to have as much pleasure as possible, try different methods and behaviours until you find what works best for you. As long as you *change something*, after all if nothing changes, nothing changes. What you change is up to you, it's YOUR strategy that will enable you to achieve your goals, not just in terms of weight loss, but in everything you want to achieve. Remember: **You don't have to wait until you achieve your desired size or shape to feel good about yourself; you can feel good about yourself NOW for no reason whatsoever!!!**

If you have the complete WLIM system listen to CD3 'Relax & Change Now'. See audio information sheet at the back of the book for more information.

If you want to attend a WLIM 'Bootcamp' weekend to experience and learn these and other techniques in person, go to the Contacts page at the back of the book.

FOOD GLORIOUS FOOD!

Any diet that brings about weight loss, does so because it causes you to eat fewer calories. Some do it by only allowing you to eat certain foods at certain times of day and not others after a certain time, others do it by restricting foods you can "combine", others by restricting one food group entirely. The High Protein diet does it by getting you to increase the amount you eat from one food group (i.e. protein) at the expense of other food groups (i.e. fat and carbohydrates), while the Low Fat diet focuses almost entirely on reducing foods that are high in fat. All of these diets have positive elements, but in most cases the baby has been thrown out with the bathwater, that is the element of the diet that is sound, is taken to extreme, sometimes to a potentially harmful extent that can put your health at risk. Few people can stick to the enforced regimes permanently so they regain the weight and more besides. Pain.

It seems crazy that in an age when we can send men to the moon, or to the depths of the sea, when we can take a heart out of one body and transplant it successfully into another body, that we haven't cracked the problem of obesity – especially when we already know the answer – **eat less and move more!**

Having stressed the importance of not eating too much, you must also look at the quality of what you eat, a fact often missed with many "fashionable diets". It is possible to lose weight and still eat really unhealthy foods: if you only ate chocolate and nothing else, but still restricted yourself to 1600 Calories per day you would lose weight. You would feel dreadful and look dreadful, although you would lose weight. With Fad Diets you cannot sustain the regime (pain) and as soon as you start eating normally again you pile the weight back on and more besides (more pain).

In my experience over the last twenty five years helping clients to lose weight, I have found that most people think of a diet as something you "go on" in the same way as you "go on" a course of antibiotics. How many times have you said to yourself or others "I am on a diet"? This assumes first of all that when you finish the diet you will come off it, and also that there are a variety of diets to choose from if that particular one doesn't work. Now you can control your inner voice and your language, you understand the importance of saying (internally in your head and externally to others) "I am a healthy eater" rather than "I am on the (bla bla) diet". Now you have mastered those skills I am going to teach you how to eat healthy foods and enjoy them without feeling like you are on a diet. That's because this isn't a diet – you are changing what you eat permanently. By the way there's only one "rule" with this system, and that is this:

IF YOU DON'T ENJOY IT – DON'T EAT IT!

I am a great believer in writing things down; from goals to appointments get it down on paper. I am not in favour of long term calorie counting – food becomes such an issue all you seem to do is weigh and measure all the time and it's a constant reminder that you are on a restriction plan, that's why I have designed the tick box system you will find later in the book which has all the benefits of keeping a food diary and non of the hassle.

As I have said several times throughout the book, honesty is important. Ask yourself now:

1.   **When do you eat?**

2.   **How much do you eat?**

When Do You Eat?
Let's deal with this first: for many overweight or fat people the problem isn't what they eat at mealtimes it's what they eat in-between that causes the weight increase. If I ask a client to write down everything they eat for a week before they come and see me, they often lose weight that week, after months of staying the same or gaining weight: they then swear blind they

only ate what they normally would eat in a week. The reality is because they had to write down everything they ate, they didn't have the chocolate bars, the crisps, the extra cheese and biscuits because they didn't want to admit to it. Without realising it, they cut out hundreds of calories they probably hadn't even acknowledged they ate.

Accepting that what you eat has made you fat is vital. Unless you have a diagnosed medical condition such as under-active thyroid or other serious metabolic disorder, you have simply eaten more than you have used. You are wearing your food.

As you might imagine, over the years I have heard all the excuses going: everything from "it's my genes" to "its my metabolism", the most common one is "I can't lose weight I don't have time to exercise or cook proper food, I only have time for fast food". If this is you **STOP** making excuses for yourself right now and take responsibility for all the times you have put food in your mouth when you didn't need it. Lets work together to find out if there is a pattern you can change. Look at the following questions:

Part 1

1. Do you eat on the run?
        Always (1) Fairly often (2) Rarely (3) Never (4)

2. Do you eat when you are not hungry
        Always (1) Fairly often (2) Rarely (3) Never (4)

3. Do you buy fast food meals
        Always (1) Fairly often (2) Rarely (3) Never (4)

4. Do you buy high fat/sugar snacks
        Always (1) Fairly often (2) Rarely (3) Never (4)

5. Do you eat for comfort
        Always (1) Fairly often (2) Rarely (3) Never (4)

6. Do you eat to relieve boredom
        Always (1) Fairly often (2) Rarely (3) Never (4)

7. Do you consume more than 2 units alcohol
        Always (1) Fairly often (2) Rarely (3) Never (4)

If you scored 35-40 CONGRATULATIONS you have a healthy approach to food and on the whole you control it, it doesn't control you.

If you scored 25-35 GOOD you are combining regular healthy choices with some less favourable choices sometimes.

If you scored 15-25 Although you are OK in some areas, in others you have work to do. Some of your behaviours are probably so instinctive you don't realise you are doing them. Look at the 1st 7 questions, any you scored a 1,2 or 3 for are key areas you need to work on. This plan will show you how to do this. In Part 2 any questions you answered 1 or 2 for also need addressing.

If you scored 10-15 DANGER! You are relying on junk food with no conscious thought as to the consequences. Not only are you overweight but you are probably undernourished, as the kinds of foods you are eating do not provide you with anything like the optimum supply of nutrients. You have the most to gain from this plan in terms of health benefits and results and in terms of weight, the most to lose. Look at the 1st 7 questions, any you scored a 1,2 or 3 for are key areas you need to work on. This plan will show you how to do this. In Part 2 any questions you answered 1 or 2 for also need addressing. You must start thinking and acting like a healthy person today and *every day* from now on. Do the visualisation and TFT exercises not just once per day, but continually throughout the day at every opportunity and last thing at night before you go to sleep. You need to change your behaviours for your own sake.

When it comes to food, eating something you don't like just because it's "good for you" is not the way to change for good. You need to genuinely enjoy your new way of eating so it will become permanent. There are enough "healthy" foods available for you to achieve your results and only eat foods you like. I keep "trying" to like olives as they are good for me, but I have now accepted I don't and never will. There are plenty of other foods that contain essential oils that I do like so it's not a problem.

I will show you exactly what you need, how much to eat and give you an easy way of balancing everything you eat using a simple colour code system. No constant weighing or measuring, just you eating foods you enjoy, that keep you satisfied *and* keep you healthy. At the end of this chapter you will find some daily record cards which are simply tick boxes: they take seconds to complete and will help you to see how healthy your diet is and what and where you need to make changes. You may find you want to carry on filling in these cards until you get the balance right automatically, or you may find that just doing it for a week or two to get you on the right track is enough. Most of my clients who achieve the greatest permanent losses fill these in for 5-6 weeks or longer, after which they can balance their diet automatically, but it's your plan so you use them for as long as you want to use them. It's a bit like learning to drive, at first you are concentrating on everything you do, wondering how you are going to remember everything at the same time, then after a while you can use the clutch, look in the mirror, turn the steering wheel etc. automatically. If you were a terrible driver and then you went on a "safe driving course" to learn how to drive well and learn new safer techniques, you would be taught new techniques and methods. It may feel different at first, but you would soon get used to your new improved skills. After a short time you wouldn't have to consciously think so much about what you are doing. This is exactly the same, it's not as if you are just going to start eating! you have been eating all your life, now you learning to eat and think about food differently, so give yourself time to learn and get used to it.

We eat food for two reasons:

1. **To give us energy to function**

2. **To give us nutrients to build and repair cells and give us health**

There are plenty of people walking around today with more energy than they need to function. All excess energy is stored as fat. You don't need me to describe what this looks like, you can imagine it as you have seen it for yourself, it may even be you. What you need and want is a balance i.e. enough energy to function at an optimal level, but also the right balance of nutrients so you not only look good you also feel great – and drastically reduce your chance of developing illness such as cancer, heart disease and other known killers. There's no need to settle for anything less.

What Are You Made Of?
Every cell is made up of the materials you provide your body with. Just like a builder using certain quality bricks and cement. The quality of the materials you use determines the quality of your cells. Put in rubbish - you are rubbish. Put in high quality foods and you get "Super Cells".

Everything you eat comes from three food groups:

CARBOHYDRATES   FATS   PROTEIN

There has been a lot of conflicting advice in the media over recent years due to the popularity of certain diets, particularly High Protein or Low Carb and I am going to start this section by giving you the correct ratios of each:

CARBS   approx 50-55%

FATS   approx 30%

PROTEINS   approx 15%

These guidelines do vary according to how active you are, for example an elite athlete may require 65% Carbs as they burn more energy, whereas a sedentary person may only need 50–55%. The same applies for Protein as athletes have more growth and repair of muscle tissue to carry out, whereas inactive individuals require less.

In order to change what you eat, you need a basic understanding of WHY you need to eat certain foods. This is not "my" diet it's just sound nutrition advice presented in a way you can understand, with a colour code formula that will help you to easily keep track of how balanced or otherwise your diet is. If it's anyone's diet – it's YOURS because you are going to choose what you eat.

Carbohydrates
As we need more carbs than either of the other two nutrients, let's start with them. What do you think carbs are? Just take a moment to mentally list the foods you class as carbs.....

My guess is that you are thinking of potatoes, rice, pasta and bread. All of these are carbohydrates as they contain glucose – which is what classifies a food as a carb, but there are many other foods that contain glucose that are not usually thought of in this group and they are - any and all fruits and vegetables. They may not contain much glucose when compared to the starchy carbs like bread and pasta, but they still come under the carbohydrate banner. To simplify it, a carb can be defined as something that grows in the soil – as opposed to coming from animal sources. Not all carbs contain the same amount of glucose and that is the key difference in their structure and is crucial when it comes to understanding weight gain and fat storage: glucose is a single molecule and because it is so small it can be absorbed directly into the blood stream. Fructose is a fruit sugar and also easily absorbed, however it varies slightly from glucose as it has two molecules and has to be taken to the liver to be separated and converted into blood sugar (glucose), before being circulated in the blood. Glucose is the body's primary source of energy. Every cell in your body requires glucose to function all of the time. No glucose – no cell function. The brain in particular has a high demand for glucose and as a result blood glucose levels have a direct influence on your mood and how you feel. The only cells in the body that can burn another source of fuel are muscle cells, and these burn a mixture of glucose and fat, but they cannot burn fat alone. **Without glucose your body cannot burn fat**.

Just to sidetrack for a moment wouldn't it be great if they could! All you would need to do to lose weight would be to go to your local gym, get on a treadmill and (providing you had the cardiovascular fitness) you could power walk or jog all day long with your muscle cells burning away all the excess fat, and get off the treadmill several pounds of fat lighter! Ah well…back to the real world..

So we know we need glucose for brain function and for energy for all cells. The problem with glucose is that it is heavy and bulky to store, so we only keep about 2000 calories in our body at any one time. It circulates in our bloodstream and is stored in small pockets in the muscle and the liver. This might sound like a lot but in fact it's only enough to maintain normal bodily functions for about 24 hours. When we have more glucose than we can store, we release excess insulin which starts a series of chain reactions that convert the excess glucose into fat and puts it in our fat cells. Unfortunately once we trigger this excess insulin release it can be a bit like using a fire extinguisher to put out a match, meaning it can be too efficient and converts not just the excess glucose but most of the circulating glucose into fat, leaving you with low blood sugar. When you have low blood sugar you are driven to eat. If I asked you now what do you eat when you think you have low blood sugar what would you say?……. I am guessing "something sweet", which perpetuates the problem and may result in another glucose high, another excess insulin release and so on and so on: you become what nutritionists often call a "sugar junkie". This can weaken your immune system and lead to constant fatigue, regular headaches, inability to concentrate, lack of coordination, inability to achieve deep restful sleep and mood swings. Sound familiar? Oh and of course – fat gain!

Converting excess glucose into fat to be stored as energy isn't necessarily a bad thing, as long as you don't convert too much.

Although you might not think of fat as being light, it is actually a very efficient way of storing billions of calories. If we stored this much energy as glucose we would be so heavy we wouldn't be able to move – however by storing it as fat, we are able to maintain an active lifestyle even if we don't like how we look.

The important principle here is that when your blood sugar is high, you go into "fat storing" mode. As with many systems the more you use this process the better your body becomes at it. You become expert fat storers! All the enzymes involved in this process get more and more efficient at storing fat, whereas the opposing enzymes that are used for burning fat become lazy and inefficient. The good news is, this process can be reversed and you can, with a healthy diet and more activity, train yourself to become expert fat burners instead of expert fat storers. Depending how long and how overweight you are. This reversal takes between a few weeks and a few months. It's certainly true that fat people find it easy to get fatter and fit people find it easier to get slimmer, as that is what their bodies are conditioned to do.

In an ideal world you would eat foods that contain enough carb to maintain normal blood sugar, but that are digested slowly, so there is a steady "trickle" of glucose into the blood, with no peaking. You can do this by understanding the Glycemic Index.

Glycemic Index (GI)
The GI was originally devised by Doctor David Jenkins in Canada, to identify foods which cause a rapid increase in blood sugar (i.e. blood glucose) in order to advise diabetics as to which to foods to eat to best maintain normal blood sugar levels. Since controlling blood sugar is important not just for diabetics, but for all of us, this approach has since been adopted and thoroughly researched by dieticians and nutritionists worldwide. At last it is being recognised in the media as a safe and effective way to plan your meals and maximise fat loss. In the GI Factor (Dr Anthony Leeds, Prof Jennie Brand Miller, Kaye Foster Powell & Stephen Coagiuri) weight loss is described as "releasing body fat" and I like that description, as that is what this plan is all about – not just losing weight on the scales but

actual fat loss and a change in body shape and size and a drastic improvement in your health. Remember the comparison earlier in the book between Arnold Schwarzenegger and Robbie Coltrane?

What is the GI?
It is quite simply a list or a chart of foods showing how quickly they release their glucose into the blood: pure glucose has a value or score of 100, whilst foods that take longer to digest have a lower score. It's as simple as that. Any foods with GI indices of greater than 70 are high GI, those with indices of 55% or less are low GI and medium GI are foods that fall in between.

Put simply, imagine a jigsaw puzzle with two pieces, its takes very little effort to break the bond between these two pieces and release the 2 single (molecules) pieces. This is what happens with table sugar, which is one molecule of glucose and one molecule of fructose bound together, your body has very little to do to separate the two molecules which then go straight into the blood stream. Compare that to a puzzle with 20 pieces, ten of which are glucose, five vitamins and five minerals, your digestive system clearly has more work to do breaking the bonds and sorting out where everything goes, so even though it technically contains more glucose than sugar, it may take longer for this glucose to be released into your blood stream as the puzzle takes longer to dismantle.

At the end of the GREEN section you will find GI tables for everyday foods, however as a general rule most white or refined foods are typically high GI. This makes sense if you think about it logically: if you think about and picture what wheat looks like as it grows naturally in a field, and then picture a slice of white bread, you realise the amount of changes the wheat goes through as it's processed. It is stripped of much of its fibre and other nutrients, this is work your digestive system would otherwise have to do, so it's much quicker to digest. If you want more information on how a low GI diet can help with a variety of medical conditions such as PCOS (Polycystic Ovary Syndrome) Insulin Resistance and Diabetes visit www.diagnosemefirst.com

Eating low GI foods makes it easy to lose weight: Research has shown that when you eat a meal with a low GI, you generally eat less than a similar meal with a high GI. As an additional benefit if you eat a low GI meal you are also less likely to overeat at your next meal. This isn't due to any "will power" simply your body responding positively to being given the right balance of foods and controlling you appetite naturally. Alternatively if you eat a lot of refined foods then you are likely to eat more calories at each meal, get hungry in between meals, and eat more at your next meal. In other words you constantly overeat. If you eat high GI foods and you want to cut down, it becomes difficult as you are constantly hungry (pain). If you eat low or medium GI foods you automatically cut down and eat less without trying (pleasure!).

The following 4 Colours Code system will help you to easily put together meals and snacks that are satisfying and that you enjoy.

COLOUR CODE PINK
Pink – starchy carbohydrates:

HIGH GI
- BREAD (wheat or any other grain)
- PASTA (wheat or corn)
- RICE
- CEREALS& GRAINS e.g. COUSCOUS
- POTATOES

LOWER GI ALTERNATIVE
- SEEDED MULTIGRAIN
- WHOLEGRAIN
- BASMATI OR BROWN
- PORRIDGE
- SWEET POTATO

The first colour on the system is PINK and it represents foods that are typically high on the GI. These foods cause a more rapid increase in blood sugar than the other colours so it's a case of eating them in moderation. There's nothing you "can't have" it's just a question of you balancing the guidelines.

I am keeping everything as simply as possible so you will need to add a pinch of common sense to the process: as you can see I have included bread in this section as most breads are very high GI, however if you choose Burgen Soya and Linseed,

Warburtons Seeded Batch or other multigrain seeded breads, they are much lower. In the same way white rice is also very high GI, with basmati being a lower alternative. Brown rice and wild rice are also lower. If you don't like brown rice a good trick is to mix fifty percent each of brown and white, which will bring the GI down. The lower GI option foods are also typically higher in fibre (which helps prevent bowel cancer and other digestive disorders) as well as other nutrients including minerals and essential fatty acids (more about this later). When it comes to potato, sweet potatoes are lower GI than white and also contain antioxidants, so again a better choice, try mashed sweet potato, you don't need to add butter just a pinch of pepper and its delicious.

I recommend for best results you restrict yourself to three (or four if you choose lower GI options) portions per day from the PINK section and that you only have one at a time: For example if you start to eat white bread before or with your meal, its high GI (as high as sugar) causes blood glucose levels to rise and once you reach the threshold of how much glucose you can carry in your blood, your body starts producing extra insulin and everything you eat after that no matter how healthy, is more likely to be converted to fat. So if you want to convert as much glucose as possible into body fat, the way to do it is to eat a plate full of pasta / potatoes / rice and have a hefty slice or two of white bread with your meal. On the other hand if you want to minimise the amount of glucose you convert to fat, have only one portion of PINK at a time and watch your portion sizes.

The reason many people didn't get the results they wanted on a traditional Low Fat Diet, is that they bulked out on many high GI foods, which although they are low in fat, e.g. bread, pasta etc, much of what they ate was high GI and the excess glucose was converted into fat, so even with low fat meals, many people still got fat or did not lose any weight at all.

PINK – PORTION SIZES

BREAD	2 THICK SLICES (use multigrain and seeded)
PASTA	1 T-CUP UNCOOKED (mix wholewheat with regular)
RICE/COUSCOUS	1 T-CUP UNCOOKED (use basmati or brown mixed)

| CEREAL | 40-60g (unrefined, avoid high sugar varieties) |
| POTATO | 1 LARGE or MAX 12oz UNCOOKED (chooose sweet potato) |

- MAX 3-4 ITEMS FROM THIS COLOUR & NOT EATEN TOGETHER UNLESS LOW GI

- RESTRICT WHEAT TO ONE PORTION PER DAY MAX (see Toxin section for explanation).

COLOUR CODE GREEN
Green – ANTIOXIDANTS (fruit and vegetables)

- Any and all fruit
- Any and all vegetables
- Beans and legumes
- Chick peas
- Soya & all vegetable derived meat alternatives

FRUITS & VEGETABLES

Fruits
All fruits contain some carbohydrate from their natural sugar content. As a general guide, tropical fruits such as melon and pineapple are slightly higher GI than temperate climate fruits such as apples pears and most citrus. The sugar contained in fruit is in the form of fructose. Unlike glucose, fructose has to go to the liver first to be converted, so whilst many fruits are deemed high in sugar, the fact it is fructose and not glucose means the sugar takes longer to be processed. One bowl of fruit salad or a banana is **not** enough to cause an excess insulin rush. Diets that advocate not eating a specific fruit for its GI are misleading. Of course if you were to eat vast amounts of fruit then you may elevate glucose levels, but you don't go into fat storage mode after one or two pieces no matter what it's GI.

Vegetables
Apart from some starchy root vegetables, most veg contain very little carbohydrate so their GI value is low. Even if you do choose

root vegetables, some of which are higher on the GI, as with fruit, one portion is **not** enough to cause an excess insulin rush and put you into fat storage mode. In simple terms ANY vegetable is a good choice either as a snack or part of a balanced meal.

Dark green veg such as spinach (great raw in a salad roll or pitta bread with lean meat in place of lettuce) broccoli and courgette are all effectively "free" when it comes to GI and can all be eaten lightly cooked, stir fried or raw in salad. Adding these to a meal can make it more filling and not only be low GI but very low in calories as well. The following tables are a guide for your information, but providing you follow the colour code guidelines you will not have to consciously try and learn the GI content of every food you eat, I have done that for you within the colour codes. Remember the aim is to keep this as simple and easy to follow as possible.

VEGETABLES

Carrots	Low
Green peas	Low
Sweetcorn	Low
Sweet potato	Low
Yam	Low
Beetroot canned	Medium
Potato – baby canned	Low
Broad beans	High
Parsnip	High
Potato	High
Pumpkin	High
Swede	High

FRUIT

Apples	Low
Bananas	Low (except when very ripe)
Berries (all)	Low
Grapefruit	Low
Grapes	Low
Mangoes	Low
Oranges	Low
Peaches	Low
Pears	Low
Plums	Low
Cantaloupe	Medium
Cherries	Medium
Kiwi	Medium
Paw Paw	Medium
Pineapple	Medium
Watermelon	High

BREAD

Chapatti	Low
Fruit loaf	Low
Granary breads	Low
Soya and linseed bread e.g. Burgen	Low
Wholegrain bread	Low
Croissant	Medium
Crumpet	Medium
Pita bread	Medium
Rye bread	Medium
Bagel	High
Wholemeal bread	High
White bread	High

BREAKFAST CEREALS

All bran	Low
Muesli	Low
Porridge oats	Low
Corn flakes	High
Instant porridge	High
Refined sugary cereals	High

MILK & DAIRY

Milk – full fat	Low
Skimmed	Low
Soya milk	Low
Yoghurt low fat	Low
Ice cream	Low
Condensed milk	Medium

BEANS PEAS & LENTILS

Baked beans	Low
Black beans	Low
Black eyed beans	Low
Borlotti beans	Low
Cannelloni beans	Low
Chick peas	Low
Haricot beans	Low
Kidney beans	Low
Lentils	Low
Lima beans	Low
Mung beans	Low
Pinto beans	Low
Romano beans	Low
Soya beans	Low
Split peas	Low

Barley	Low
Buckwheat	Low
Bulgar	Low
Noodles	Low
Pasta dried/fresh	Low
Quinoa	Low
Arborio rice	Low
Basmati	Medium
Wild rice	Medium
Instant rice	High
Jasmine rice	High
Canned spaghetti	High

Knowing that some carbs can help keep you full and automatically eat less, is a great reason to eat them, but there are even more good reasons to include them in your diet. Many carbs (in fact pretty much all carbs apart from refined carbs and sugar) contain precious substances called antioxidants. I am not going to get too technical here but I do want to show you how valuable these substances are and what they do: here's the science!

Within all molecules are electrons. These electrons like to work in pairs. When all electrons have a pair, or partner the molecule is stable. Stable is good. See Fig 1.

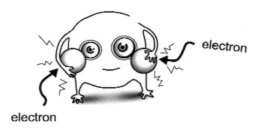

electron

electron

Fig 1. A happy, well-balanced human cell

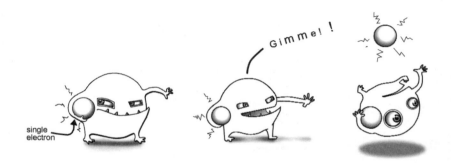

Fig 2. Free radical

If there is only one electron i.e. it is unpaired, it is a called a **free radical**. These free radicals do not like only having one electron and go around the body trying to pair off with another electron. They do this by breaking into the structure of healthy cells and stealing one of its electrons. This leaves the previously healthy cell, unhealthy. Once that cell is damaged it can have a domino effect as more and more free radicals are created and more cells damaged. Free radicals cause cancer, heart disease, many other degenerative disease, and prematurely age cells, including skin cells. They are bad bad bad. See Fig 2.

There are naturally occurring substances in foods called ANTIOXIDANTS. These are super efficient substances that eliminate free radicals. These include Vitamins A C and E as well as minerals such as selenium. These vital nutrients are found in fresh unprocessed carbs, such as fruit, vegetables, whole-grains and some essential fatty acids. This is good, but once the antioxidant has bonded with a free radical, it cannot do anything else; whereas it would normally have a variety of other important roles to play such as strengthening the immune system, or making collagen and other substances including hormones. It can perform none of these tasks if it is used up combating free radicals (see Fig. 3).

Almost all your daily requirement of VC is used up combating the free radicals contained in just one cigarette.

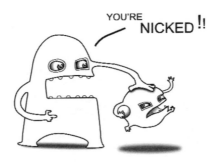

Fig 3. Antioxidant

You don't have to be an expert to learn which foods contain antioxidants; there is a very simple guideline:

If it's fresh and colourful – it contains antioxidants

The good news is that foods that contain antioxidants are typically low GI. For example sweet potatoes are much lower on the GI than white potatoes and are rich in antioxidants. Other foods high in antioxidants include:

Carrots	Peppers (all colours)	Spinach
Broccoli	Watercress	Peas
Cabbage	Cauliflower	Tomatoes
All berries, e.g. strawberries, cranberries	Melon	Lemons
Mangoes	Pumpkin	Kiwi fruit
Oranges	Avocados	Oily fish
Wheatgerm	Fresh seeds	Fresh nuts

Have at least six portions of antioxidants every day. In this way you will automatically be eating all the antioxidants and fibre you need and not only reducing your risk of cancer and other diseases but boosting your energy levels, improving your skin, hair, nails and concentration levels as well as losing weight. There are many antioxidant supplements on the market. I recommend 'Zambroza', a delicious exotic fruit drink (see back of book for details).

Eating six or more portions of **GREEN** is easy to do if you plan ahead, but not so easy if you leave it till evening and then face 6 oranges or apples! Aim for two portions per meal. For example have a glass of fruit juice with breakfast and if you are having cereal chop some fruit and put it on top, with a handful of seeds. If you are having toast have a piece of fruit as well afterwards, or some fruit in a yoghurt. For lunch if you are having a sandwich or stuffed pitta bread have a handful of watercress or spinach, or have a bowl of fresh salad (see recipe suggestions) with some meat or fish. With your main meal have at least two portions of antioxidants in the form of vegetables or salad with the main course or have a fruit salad as a dessert.

Foods that are shown in green colour but with ★ are carbs that are also good vegetarian sources of protein. If you are a vegetarian you should include these foods in your daily intake.

I have found most people fall into one of two categories when it comes to cooking meals: the first type (like me) are one pot chefs, things like stir fry's, curries, stews etc. and the second the more traditional meat, potatoes and veg on the plate separately (like my parents). Neither one is better than the other it's just a question of doing what you like. If you are a one pot cook, instead of making chicken curry make a chicken and vegetable curry, or instead of a beef stir fry make a beef and vegetable stir fry (anything sprouting such as bean sprouts are nutritionally good), or if you prefer to serve a pork chop with new potatoes and carrots, simply add another vegetable as well.

Carbohydrates contain only 4 calories per gram, as opposed to fat which contains 9 calories per gram. This means taking out some of the high fat foods and replacing them with low GI carbs can have a dramatic impact on your total calorific intake, without you having to eat less food – just different foods. In fact you can have more weight of food on your plate and still eat fewer calories and feel more satisfied.

You will find some great recipes in this book to get you started, but aim to design your own personal diet that you really enjoy and that fits in with your lifestyle.

GREEN – PORTION SIZES

ANY FRUIT = 1 PIECE (except avocado = $\frac{1}{2}$ and also contains EFAs)

FRUIT JUICE = 250 ml

VEGETABLES = EQUIVALENT 1 MUG

LENTILS/BEANS/CHICK PEAS ★ = 1 CUP UNCOOKED

PER DAY: 3 X FRUIT & 3-6 X VEG

★ Vegetarians have at least 2 of these daily

COLOUR CODE BLUE
Green – Fat and Protein

- All types of meat
- All dairy products e.g. milk, cheese (except ice cream or cream)
- All fish
- Fresh nuts and seeds
- Oils e.g. olive oil
- Butter /peanut butter

To keep it simple I have combined Fat and Protein into one colour, **BLUE** for you. This is because with the exception of pure fats such as butter or oils, you will typically find foods that contain protein contain fat and vice-versa.

FATS

Fats get a bad press and that is half way correct, as certain types of fat not only cause you to gain weight but increase your risk of heart disease cancer and many other illness. On the other hand other "good" fats actually decrease your risk of disease, contain valuable antioxidants and actually help you metabolise fat and lose weight. The two different types of fat are:

Saturated Fat

Saturated simply means SOLID at body temperature (i.e. 37°). If you are eating foods that contain saturated fat then no matter what consistency or texture they are when you eat them, when they adopt your body temperature they solidify. They are not as solid as set cement, they are more like runny candle wax, sticky and gooey. Even saturated fats aren't all bad, they are important for insulating and protecting our organs and for energy; however it's very easy to store far more energy than you are ever going to need, which is what your body has already been doing if you are fat.

In the UK over the last two years there has been a television advert designed at encouraging smokers to stop smoking: It shows a cigarette being unrolled, and instead of tobacco, the inside is a sticky gooey dirty white substance that drips slowly out the end – representing saturated fat. It's disgusting to look at, if food looked like this when you were eating it you would probably not bother. Maybe you have gone into the kitchen sometime after cooking a roast dinner, or sausages or other fatty meat, and found the bottom of the pan covered in sticky white fat. Because the room temperature is lower than cooking temperature, as the fat cools it solidifies, and what you see in the pan is exactly the same as what is happening inside your body: your blood vessels will be full of this sticky white fat which the body converts into *your* body fat (as opposed to the animals body fat – which is really whose fat you are eating) by putting it into your fat cells.

Unfortunately foods high in saturated fat such as pies and chips look much more appetising than sticky white goo, so it's hard to make the immediate connection: that comes later when you can't get in your clothes (pain) and you have already eaten it. Ice cream may not look like animal fat – but what do you think gives it is texture? Whipped ice creams are often made with pig fat – doesn't that sound appetising? Cold pig fat mixed with sugar and flavouring – "yum yum". Just visualise that image next time someone offers you an ice cream! However there are better alternatives, for example Solero are made with skimmed milk, as are some low fat frozen yoghurts, so you can still enjoy a healthier version of the original and not gain fat (pleasure).

- Saturated fat comes exclusively from animal sources with only two exceptions, which are

- Coconut oil (believed to have some health benefits if consumed in moderation).

- Palm oil (used in sweets to make them sticky).

Reducing your intake of animal products, not just meat, is a good way to not only reduce calories, but also reduce fat intake. If you are a meat eater then 4-6oz for women and 6-8oz for men is a normal portion size (based on a moderately active adult). If you eat cheese then aim for 2-3 oz of hard cheese as a portion, which can be slightly increased for soft cheese such as brie to 3-4oz.

I am not recommending you become a total vegetarian, although a vegetarian diet can be extremely healthy if followed correctly, what I am suggesting is that you restrict the amount of most animal products In your diet, excluding oily fish which are extremely healthy (providing they are not farmed).

There are obvious unhealthy high fat meals such as chicken korma, but it doesn't mean stop eating Indian food altogether – if you are out or even having a take away as long as its not an everyday occurrence you can still enjoy these types of foods *sometimes* and lose weight: for example in an Indian restaurant choose tomato based sauces instead of the kormas and masalas, and ask your waiter for it to be cooked in as little fat as possible, or choose tandoori dishes. Bear in mind one naan bread is up to 500 Cal. Chinese meals are also typically very high but there are some dishes that offer damage limitation such as steamed fish in black bean sauce. Any fried rice (Indian or Chinese) is going to contain a lot more calories than plain rice so that's a really easy way to save calories and reduce fat. It's hard to get a low fat variety of fish and chips from a chip shop so go for much smaller portions, or get oven baked varieties you can do at home.

Unsaturated Fat
These fats are liquid at body temperature. They are used for

growth and repair. Importantly every cell in your body is made up of Essential fatty Acids (EFA's) which are used to make the cell membrane. This membrane – or cell wall has to be permeable, which means it has to allow things to pass through either to get nutrients into the cell or waste products out. It also has to repel free radicals and attacks from viruses and bacteria. Cells made from sub standard fats cannot do this and that is one of the reasons they increase your risk of cancer and other life threatening and debilitating diseases.

Unsaturated Fatty Acids (UFA's) don't stick together in the blood like Saturated Fatty Acids (SFA's) making them less likely to cause blood clots.

Symptoms of deficiency of EFA's include the following:

- High blood pressure

- PMS or breast pain

- Eczema or dry skin

- Dry eyes

- Inflammatory conditions such as arthritis

- Water retention

- Tingling in arms and legs

- Prone to infection

- Decline in memory or learning ability

- Lack of coordination

- Impaired vision

- Poor fat metabolism and digestion

UFAs can be broken into Monounsaturated Fatty Acids (MUFA's) and Polyunsaturated Fatty Acids (PUFA's), including Omega 3 and Omega 6, all of which are extremely healthy. The body can use MUFA's and change the length of the fatty acid chain to make other fatty acid chains for a variety of specific purposes: Omega 3 and Omega 6 however are ESSENTIAL which means the body CANNOT manufacture them therefore they must be eaten.

An added benefit of EFA's is that they help with metabolism and therefore aid fat loss. The ironic fact is that in the Western World we typically eat a diet too high in fat (research suggests we consume in excess of 40-45% on average) but are deficient in EFA's. In other words we eat the wrong fats.

The following table shows the fats we should be including in our diet:

Monounsaturated Fats	Omega 6 (Linoleic Acid)	Omega 3 (Linolenic Acid)
Olives / olive oil	Soyabean	Flaxseed (linseed)
Canola oil	Safflower	Soyabean
Almond oil	Sunflower	Rapeseed (canola)
Avocado	Corn	Pumpkin
	Wheatgerm	Walnut
	Sesame	Fish
	Evening Primrose Oil	

Include at least two of the following foods in your diet every day for maximum health and fat loss:

• Fresh seeds (especially hemp) -1 dessert spoonful

• Fresh nuts e.g. Brazil nuts - 8 nuts per day

- Olives – 6-8

- Oily fish - anything with teeth but NOT farmed fish (which often do not contain EFA) , organic or wild only

- Fresh oil e.g. olive oil –1 spoonful on salads / dressings or in stir-fry

- Avocado (green)

- Whole unprocessed grains

Avocados are a great source of monounsaturated fats (the same oil as fresh olives) and though traditionally viewed as a "sin" on many diets, I encourage you to have a portion (1/2 avocado) as a sandwich filler or in salads or just mashed on multigrain toast (lovely!) as they also contain a substance which suppresses appetite and are low on the GI.

Fats are combined with Proteins to make the colour **BLUE** in the colour code system:

PROTEIN
Protein is a vital component of our diet, and there has been a lot of controversy in recent years as to the benefits or otherwise of the "High Protein" or "Low Carb" Diets, and the many other diets that are variations on the same theme.

There are a few fundamental differences in how the body handles protein when compared to fat or carb: protein takes a long time to digest and therefore keeps us satisfied for a long time. It does not in itself contain glucose therefore has no GI score. Whereas carb digestion begins in the mouth, protein can only be digested in the stomach as it is much harder to break down. The stomach is a sealed sack that contains a special acid (called hydrochloric acid) which is required to break down protein. The stomach lining is covered in a coating of thick phlegm like fluid that protects it against the harmful effects of the acid. If it does escape to other areas outside the stomach it causes burns and ulcers, so there are valves at the entrance and exit to prevent this from happening.

Protein contains nitrogen, which the body converts into ammonia and then urea which is excreted by the kidneys. This highly acidic process can be undertaken safely all the time the correct amount of protein is being eaten, however if the diet is consistently high in protein then the kidneys begin to suffer from the effects of the extra work they are having to do. This can be anything from slight back ache, to potential kidney failure. There are other negative effects of a long term high protein diet, for example the body becomes too acidic. To combat this it takes calcium out of the bones which is very alkaline and dumps it into the bloodstream to compensate. This can lead to osteoporosis as well as increased risk of heart disease. One of the biggest disadvantages with High Protein type diets is that they prohibit the intake of fruits and veg as well as the high GI refined carbs. As we have discussed these foods contain valuable antioxidants, so not only are you putting your body at risk of disease, but you are denying yourself the nutrients that protect against these diseases. That's throwing the baby out with the bathwater. Not good.

Having explained the down side to a High Protein diet, it's important to stress that protein IS a vital nutrient and should make up approximately 15-20% of your total intake, as it is a vital component of ALL living cells. After water it is the most abundant nutrient in our body. The reason you need less protein than carb or fat is that unlike the other two it is not used for energy production, therefore doesn't need to be replaced as often, as not as much is used up.

Having protein with your meal helps keep you full not just when you eat, but until the next meal, so you are less likely to snack.

If you are a vegetarian then you need to ensure you consume vegetables and grains that are high in good quality protein such as:

• Quinoa (a grain/fruit from South America)

- Soya (e.g. Tofu)

- Beans

- Lentils

- Fresh seeds

- Fresh nuts

- Wholegrains

- Low fat dairy products

BLUE – PORTION SIZES

MEAT OR FISH = 6-8oz
OIL = 1 TSP
SEEDS = 1 DESERT SPOON
FRESH NUTS = 8 NUTS
MILK (SEMI-SKIMMED OR SKIMMED) = 250ml
BUTTER/PEANUT BUTTER = $1/_2$ oz (THIN SCRAPE FOR 2 SLICES)
CHEESE = 2-3 oz hard or 3-4oz soft (cottage cheese 1 small carton)

PER DAY: MAX 5 ITEMS AS LISTED
- Have at least 1 item from this section or the GREEN ★ section
  with each meal to keep you satisfied.

You will find that the portion sizes vary for BLUE foods more than any other. This is because you may have a pork chop or a steak counting as one portion, and a yoghurt or 2-3oz cheese as another. In this way you need to use your common sense. I am working on the basis that you will have no more than one portion of meat per day and the rest come from dairy or vegetarian sources, such as nuts and seeds.

If you include the right amount of protein in your diet you will naturally eat less. If you know you are not going to eat for some time, have a protein based meal with something from the green section. For example beans or poached eggs on toast are great low GI meals. If you are in a rush or don't like a large breakfast then I recommend SynerProtein, which is a formulated drink, free from milk, eggs or any animal derivatives. It is an excellent source of protein which you mix with water and comes in various flavours. It can also be used in a blender to add to smoothies. For more information and how to order it see the contact details at the back of the book.

COLOUR CODE RED

- All sweets & confectionary e.g. chocolate toffee etc
- Ice cream/cream
- Alcohol
- Crisps
- Pies and pastries – sweet/savory
- Sugar
- Instant gravy granules or sauces
- Carbonated drinks
- High fat snacks e.g. sausage rolls
- Meringues
- Anything from a packet box or jar not shown elsewhere in the charts
- Fish and chips or similar
- Anything you KNOW is unhealthy but isn't on this list

PER DAY: MAX 250 CAL (NOT COMPULSORY!)

Most of the foods we have discussed so far have health benefits; however being only human it is nice to be able to have something that is unhealthy – just because you like it – every now and then. In fact in my experience it's essential to know that "you can if you want to" to stay out of the "diet" mentality. For this reason I suggest a guideline of between 200-250 Calories per day ONLY IF YOU WANT THEM of anything unhealthy (food or drink!). It is important you keep track of just how much of these foods you eat and for that reason they are included in the daily tick boxes as RED. Unhealthy foods generally come in packets that tell you their calorific content so it's not difficult to monitor. If you are having fish and chips or an Indian meal it can be anything between 2000 and 3000 calories or sometimes more, so when you are out I recommend you adopt a *damage limitation policy*: this means monitoring what else you have that day closely, or having smaller portions and less often. If I am out for a three course meal I usually choose a healthy(ish) starter such as home made soup or smoked salmon or salad, as opposed to a high fat paté or garlic mushrooms dripping in butter. I will have a lean piece of meat in a non creamy sauce, or fish, and new or jacket potatoes and vegetables for main course. When it comes to dessert I will enjoy a bowl of profiteroles or some cheesecake, safe in the knowledge that I don't do it everyday and everything is OK in moderation. If you are not a sweet lover you can go for the high fat starter or main and compromise on the other two. Whatever works for you, so you enjoy the meal and still feel like you are in control and you are not going to feel "guilty" the next day.

Bear in mind these RED calories are NOT COMPULSORY. With the mind exercises and the new memory programmes you have learnt and are continuing to learn, you may find you do not want these foods at all. When you associate pleasure with **not** eating them and **PAIN** when you do, it becomes easy to not eat foods that you know make you fat (pain).

Sometimes when people offer me a 2nd helping of something, or an extra large pudding, I just think "I want to be slim more than I want to eat extra pudding". Just maintain control of your inner chatter and be honest with yourself.

TOXINS
There are substances that are known to be toxic to everyone, such as mercury, lead and most heavy metals. There are also substances that certain individuals are allergic to, which can be anything from fish, nuts, bananas, or any foods that are healthy and nutritious for other people. Then there are foods or substances that are individual energy toxins (IETs). Although IETs don't cause an immediate allergic response, they sap your body of energy, cause fatigue, headaches, insomnia and contribute to a range of health and emotional problems, in

particular anxiety, depression and compulsive disorders. IETs also contribute to weight gain for a number of reasons: they cause fluid retention and bloating, they interfere with our body's ability to control hunger and cause cravings and they make you so tired that you become less active.

IBS is a widely recognised condition which can be caused by IETs. Elimination of the offending food can result in almost immediate and rapid weight loss and restoration of energy levels and vitality.

The most common IETs are usually the things you consume most of. Bearing that in mind, wheat and dairy are often the worst offenders.

IETs are not a new phenomena, Dr Arthur F Coca MD was researching the effects of IETs on health in the 1950's and devised a test that can be done by individuals at home:

1.   sit down comfortably and take your pulse rate for a
      full minute

2.   stand up and take pulse rate again for a full minute.

If the pulse rate increases by more than 10 beats it indicates your body is being stressed by IETs.

Over the last few decades Dr Roger Callahan, founder of TFT has devoted much of his time to researching these toxins, how to diagnose them and how to treat them. Traditionally this is done with a TFT practitioner using kinesiology or muscle testing. It can also be done using voice analysis. This system is called Voice Technology (VT). Analysing your voice can identify changes in voice patterns that pinpoint which foods or substances are IETs for you. This can be done quickly and easily over the telephone and is the most accurate and cost effective method of identifying IETs. It is a highly specialized process and only a dozen or so people in the world have been trained to this level. For more details see the Contacts page at the back of the book.

Common symptoms of IETs

- general malaise
- food cravings
- negative emotions for no reason
- anxiety
- lack of motivation
- panic attacks
- bloating
- stress
- headaches
- diarrhea
- emotional and physical weakness
- weight gain
- obsessive compulsive disorder

If you would like more information on VT and how to test for IETs there is a contact email at the back of the book (pg 149).

ACID / ALKALINE BALANCE IN THE BODY

For good health it is essential to maintain a healthy pH in the body and a healthy diet contributes to this. The pH scale ranges from 0-14. A pH of 7 is neutral.

Substances with a pH higher than 7 are alkaline and substances with a pH of less than 7 are acidic. The difference between each point i.e. a pH of 6 and a pH of 7 is 10 times. Bearing this in mind it's easy to understand why even a slight shift in pH can make a significant difference, whether it's positive or negative.

A healthy body is slightly alkaline with an optimum pH of 7.365 for blood and 7.4 for spinal fluid and saliva.

Problems associated with acidic pH:

- heightened risk of infection from bacteria
- heightened risk of infection from yeast
- heightened risk of infection from parasites

- heightened risk of infection from viruses
- heightened risk of cancer
- arthritis
- heart disease
- many degenerative conditions
- excessive fatigue
- digestive problems
- kidney problems
- osteoporosis

The body maintains homeostatic pH by depositing and withdrawing alkaline minerals such as calcium from body tissues such as bone. If a diet is highly acidic (typically a high protein diet) then calcium is leeched from the bones and put into the blood in order to restore homeostasis: this puts incredible strain on the kidneys which filter the blood and also increases the risk of cardiovascular and associated diseases as the blood becomes more viscous.

To determine if a food is acid or alkaline, it is burned and the ash (which contains the minerals within the food) is mixed with water and then analysed.

Digestion works in much the same way. Instead of heat and flames, enzymes operating at low temperatures "burn" the food. The residual minerals are either acidic or alkaline depending on the food. A lemon, for example, leaves a residual alkaline ash consisting of minerals salts such as sodium, potassium and calcium: So while a lemon will taste acidic and have an acid pH if tested prior to digestion, after digestion its ash will be alkaline and so will its effect on the body. Hot water with a slice of lemon is a great alkaline drink.

Proteins on the other hand leave an acidic ash. The net effect of protein consumption, (whether from animal or vegetable sources), is to increase acidity.

Diets which are high in protein, fat and carbohydrates and low in greens and raw food, are primarily acidic and as a result stress the digestive mechanisms and overload the immune system. These kinds of diets are made worse by the typically high intake of processed foods containing food additives, pesticides and stimulating foods such as caffeine, that are common in the Western diet. In an attempt to solve the problem of worsening public water quality, more and more people are turning to water in plastic bottles and containers. What is usually not realized is that virtually all bottled water is highly acidic and missing the essential alkalizing minerals. A good water filter is often a better option. I strongly recommend an alkaline drink daily. My personal favourite is Natures Sunshine Liquid Chlorophyll details of which can be found at the back of the book on the "recommended products" page. It works like squash in that you simply add the concentrate to water and drink it as a refreshing drink. It is also a natural detoxifier mild antibiotic and deodorizer so freshens breath as well as being alkaline.

Examples of Common Food Types that have a Strongly Acid pH (avoid)	Examples of Common Food Types that are Mildly Acidic	Examples of Common Food Types that are Mildly Alkaline	Examples of Common Food Types that are Strongly Alkaline (Best)
red meat	grains	tofu	Soy
alcohol	legumes	vegetables	vegetables
eggs	most nuts	olive oil	Real salt
dried fruit	canola oil	goat milk	sprouts
sugars	fruit juice	almonds	garlic
hard cheese	milk, rice/ soy milk	buckwheat	alkaline water

You can find out more information about the effects of acidic foods and also information on water purifiers at www.ionizers.org

You will notice that the two week quick start detox programme has a strong emphasis on alkaline foods. When you follow the colour code charts you will be maximising alkaline foods and minimising acidic foods automatically. Not only will you be losing weight but you may also slow down the ageing process and drastically reduce your risk of disease.

Daily check cards

This card system is to enable you to keep track of what you are learning and eating in a simple easy to manage way. You simply tick the box when you have had a portion (as stated in the portion size box shown in each section) and when all the boxes for that colour have been ticked, you know anything you eat over and above that is more than you need. Simply photocopy the cards on the last page of the book, or make your own along these lines. If you have the WLIM system you will find a printable version on your Resource CD, along with 28 days worth of recipes and ideas.

IT'S YOUR MOVE

I am often asked "What is the best exercise for fat loss?", the honest answer is, "Not necessarily the one that burns most calories (which by the way is cross country ski-ing!) but the one that *you* will actually do". Whether you join a local club (always a good idea as you will get the expertise and the support you need) or follow your own plan, as long as you do it regularly you will be burning calories you otherwise would have stored as fat.

If you are overweight or overfat, you need to burn more calories as well as take less in. Eat Less *and* Move More.

There are two aspects to exercise for weight loss

1.   **Aerobic** exercise e.g. fast walking, cycling etc

2.   **Resistance** strength or toning exercises using some kind of resistance e.g. gym programme

BOTH ARE VITAL FOR FAT LOSS

Your body has a constant need for oxygen. You cannot live without it – therefore it stands to reason that the more efficient you are at pumping oxygen through your body the "fitter" you will be. Aerobic simply means "with oxygen" its not a fancy or a technical term used for a specific activity or exercise, in fact we are "working" aerobically all the time just surviving: so for the purposes of this section when I use the term "working aerobically" I mean your heart is working harder than it does when you are at rest.

As we go about our passive existence (without exercise) most of our energy needs are met from the glucose we derive from carbohydrates. A little fat is burnt but not much compared to how much fat you store.

Glucose and fat are two separate energy stores within the body – glucose is like a current account, where the funds are easily accessible and fat is like a deposit account which you have to dip into to top up when funds in the current account are too low. Unfortunately, as I mentioned earlier in the book **YOU CANNOT BURN FAT WITHOUT GLUCOSE,** in fact if your glucose levels are too low then it actually makes it harder to burn fat, as you will feel extremely tired and heavy legged and probably unable to exercise to any significant intensity anyway.

Bit of a shame that! Otherwise you could set off on your jog in the morning and (providing your heart was strong enough to keep you going) carry on all day using up your fat stores as fuel, and end the day be a dress size or two smaller! That would be the ultimate quick start plan wouldn't it! But, like most things that sound to good to be true – it is.

So we are faced with the fact that we need to be more active to use more fat.

AEROBIC EXERCISE MEANS USING MORE OXYGEN
When you start to do aerobic exercise you burn glucose more quickly than when you are being passive: your brain detects this change and starts to release more fat (in the form of triglycerides or TG's) into the blood to be carried to the muscles. This fat then mixes with the glucose to make the glucose last longer. A simple comparison would be to water down a strong drink to make it go further. Instead of relying on mainly glucose with a small amount of fat, you begin to drastically change the ratio in favor of burning more fat and less glucose.

As you are burning more energy more quickly your metabolic rate goes up. All the time your metabolic rate stays elevated you are burning more calories – and the good news is that it can stay elevated for over ten hours after you finished exercising, depending on how hard you worked. You don't have to go flat out for this benefit, as long as you feel challenged (though not absolutely shattered) after your work out, you have done enough to burn extra calories for hours afterwards. If you exercise three times per week for an hour, this can snowball into

30 hours of extra calorie burning.

STRONG MUSCLES BURN MORE FAT
The amount of muscle tissue you have on your body determines to a large extent the amount of calories you burn. 1lb muscle burns approximately 40 calories per day at rest. If over time you lose 5lbs of muscle tissue through inactivity, then you burn 200 Calories less per day. If you eat the same amount of food as before you lost the muscle, then you gain weight even without consuming an extra calorie.

The good news if you have lost muscle tissue, is that its reversible. Simply by toning and strengthening your muscles you can re-train them to burn more fat and completely change your shape. Ideally this is best done in a gym environment – but don't panic if you don't feel ready for that just yet, ANYTHING IS BETTER THAN NOTHING!

HOW FIT ARE YOU?
In the same way as I recommend taking a good look at your current diet so you know exactly what you need to change – a simple fitness test can be a bit of an eye opener as to how fit or unfit you are. This one can be done easily at home. Common sense dictates that if you have any health problems, in particular respiratory problems, that you have a full medical check up before undertaking any form of exercise – even this simple fitness test.

STEP TEST (source: Canadian Public Health Association Project)
Using a 12 inch step or stair (or as near to this as possible e.g. bottom stair).

Step on and off for 3 minutes:

Step up with one foot, then up with the other, then down with the first and down with the second. Change the lead leg several times without changing the tempo. It is important to maintain a steady tempo throughout – if you have a metronome that would be perfect! Alternatively find a record with a steady beat of approx 122 beats per minute or thereabouts to guide you.

When you have completed the three minutes, remain standing whilst you take your pulse.

To take your pulse place your 2 middle fingers to the corner of your lips and smile, keeping your fingers traveling in a straight vertical line slide them down under your chin and press into your neck just above your voice box or 1-2 inches down your neck, roll your fingers in towards your windpipe and press gently. Practice this a few times before you start the test. It is much easier to feel your pulse when you have been exercising.

Compare your result to the charts below:

WOMEN

AGE	18-25	26-35	36-45	46-55-	56-65	65+
Excellent	<85	<88	<90	<94	<95	<90
Good	85-98	88-99	90-102	94-104	95-104	90-102
Above average	99-108	100-111	103-110	105-115	105-112	103-115
Average	109-117	112-119	111-118	116-120	113-118	116-122
Below Average	118-126	120-126	119-128	121-129	119-128	123-128
Poor	127-140	127-138	129-140	130-135	129-139	129-134
Very Poor	>140	>138	>140	>135	>139	>134

MEN

AGE	18-25	26-35	36-45	46-55-	56-65	65+
Excellent	<79	<81	<83	<87	<86	<88
Good	79-89	81-89	83-96	87-97	86-97	88-96
Above average	90-99	90-99	97-103	98-105	98-103	97-103
Average	100-105	100-107	104-112	106-116	104-112	104-113
Below Average	106-116	108-117	113-119	117-122	113-120	114-120
Poor	117-128	118-128	120-130	123-132	121-129	121-130
Very Poor	>128	>128	>130	>132	>129	>130

You don't have to enjoy exercise to benefit from it. Up until recently I had a large dog who I walked or ran with everyday, whatever the weather or however busy I was I HAD to find or make time, even if it was only a quick 20 min walk, to take him out. Since I lost him, it's much harder to motivate myself to get out, but I want to be slim more than I don't want to exercise, so I motivate myself to go out 3 times per week. Sometimes if I am out power walking or running and it's a beautiful day I really enjoy it, but on grey days it's not so much fun! So I put on my ipod and I go anyway because I want to be slim. It's a choice. You have exactly the same choices. Start associating pleasure with exercising, even if it's just the sense of achievement you get when its over! And pain with not exercising as that means staying fat. We talked earlier in the book about values and beliefs, go back and re-read this section before you start your regime and model a plan that's right for you.

Work on the basis ANYTHING IS BETTER THAN NOTHING. Start with some aerobic work which may be anything from walking to running, cycling or skipping. If you want a cheap easy to store piece of equipment for home, get a rebounder. Simply bounce, jog or power march on it whilst watching tv. Rebounding has been shown to improve lymph circulation so has added benefits and can easily be stored under the bed (for more details see information at the back of the book). Take your score from the fitness test tables and using the following guidelines in the PRE scale below aim to work out aerobically at least 3-4 times per week.

If you have the complete WLIM system a full 28 day workout is available on the 'Resource CD', perfect to get you started to build on an existing regime.

"Below Average" or less, 5-10 minute intervals at level 4-5 on the PRE scale

"Average" 10-15 minutes at level 6

"Above Average" 15-17 minutes at level 6-7

"Good" 20+ mins at level 7

"Excellent" 30+ minutes at level 8

The Perceived Rate Of Exertion Scale is a quick and easy way for you to see how hard you are working. Simply look at the numbers and compare them with how you feel when you are exercising.

PERCEIVED RATE OF EXERTION (PRE) SCALE

No.	How You Should Feel
1.	No effort at all
2.	Slight effort
3.	Some effort
4.	Rate of breathing starts to increase & deepen
5.	Slightly breathless able to speak quite freely, i.e. brief chat, some perspiration
6.	Breathless but comfortable able to speak but shorter paragraphs, perspiring
7.	More breathless able to speak in shorter sentences, freely perspiring
8.	Quite breathless, able to speak a few words, perspiring freely
9.	Very breathless, only able to speak briefly, feel heart rate pumping
10.	Really breathless, struggling to continue, unable to speak at all

Aim to exercise at least 3–4 times per week. For best results become more active everyday in everything you do.

QUICK START TWO WEEK ENERGY BOOSTING DETOX

Nothing motivates us more than seeing results quickly. That's exactly why I have designed this 2 *week energy boosting detox plan* to give you a real head start. It would be impractical to stay on this exact plan permanently, so it is just a healthy boost you can use whenever you need it. You will probably lose more weight on this plan than you normally do in a two week period (sometimes as much as 10lbs) so please expect the rate of weight loss to slow down somewhat when you design your own long term plan based on the colour code system. Normally a loss of 1-2 lbs a week of body fat is enough to lose a dress size every 4-6 weeks. With some "diets" the actual loss in terms of weight is greater, but much of it is fluid and less or none of it fat so your shape doesn't change. With this plan, particularly if you exercise regularly, its actual body fat that's lost and your shape can change dramatically.

With this 2 week plan I have done all the colour coding and calorie counting for you so it couldn't be simpler – all you have to do is follow it by choosing the foods you like. You don't need to write down what you eat or even do the tick sheets as long as you are sticking to the recipes and meal choices suggested. However they are designed to make it easy for you – so you decide.

I must stress again that whilst this can be a great start now, and at times a boost to progress, taking a long-term view of what you eat is the only way to get long- term results. Many of my clients do this 2 week plan every 3-4 months and others just once a year. It really is up to you. It is a bit like an intensive course in eating a healthy diet, so whilst it will be great for some it is by no means a compulsory part of the overall programme, which is designed to help you make permanent changes. I have included some herbal supplements which maximise the effectiveness of the plan both in terms of weight loss and detoxifying, details of which are on the "recommended products" page at the back of the book, however if you would rather just follow the guidelines without these they are by no means compulsory.

HOW DOES IT WORK?
There are five main aims of the detox:

1. **To cleanse your body and in particular your digestive system**

2. **To motivate your bowels to open regularly (essential for weight loss and health)**

3. **To maximise antioxidant intake**

4. **To balance pH**

5. **To lose weight**

As you will have realised by now I do not recommend faddy diets. This plan is ideal for short term but is quite strict and parts of it would be harder to maintain in the long term so you will find 2 weeks just right. As with any "diet" you need to control your intake i.e. how many calories you eat and balance this with your outgoing energy i.e. how many calories you burn. Because so much of this 2-week plan is based on fresh foods such as fruits and vegetables, which are typically very low calorie foods – you may actually feel you you are eating more than you normally do – when in fact you are not. It is important not to go below the threshold of 1500 Calories per day for women and 2000 for men, as this can lead to muscle loss rather than fat loss, which is not what we want! At the same time do not exceed 1800 calories for women and 2300 for men. I have done all the calculations for you all you need to do is follow the guidelines.

In addition to the foods I recommend taking a "Healthy Starter Pack" from Natures Sunshine. This is in tablet form to be taken along with regular meals and will help clear toxins from the body, improve elimination, expel parasites, detoxify the kidneys and the liver, purify the blood and cleanse the whole body of cellular waste. Details are on the "recommended products" page at the back of the book.

Many people who are overweight do not open their bowels very often. This leads not only to weight gain but also to toxicity and can contribute to feeling tired all the times, headaches as well as poor skin and many other unpleasant conditions. It also increases your chance of suffering bowel cancer. Take one of each tablet with the evening meal once per day for the first 3-5 days, then increase to 2 of each tablet. You will notice on 2 tablets that things really start moving! If you are comfortable on 2 tablets you can increase to 3. If not stay on 2 tablets, which means the herbal course will continue for longer than the 14 days. This is absolutely fine, just continue taking them with meals until the course is finished. Detailed instructions are on the box.

The plan itself is packed full of foods that are rich in nutrients and alkaline, so it helps de-toxify and balance the body and boost your energy levels. There is sufficient protein (lean low fat sources) to stabilise hunger and leave you satisfied, particularly if you use the SynerProtein. A word of caution – because we are eliminating all foods that contain additives for much of the 2 weeks you may feel lethargic or experience headaches if you do not prepare properly. The first few days its crucial to *gradually* reduce foods such as tea coffee sugar and alcohol. **Where possible take a week prior to the detox to gradually eliminate tea and coffee so that you are clear of these before you start**. This and drinking plenty of fresh juice and or water will help you to feel energised throughout the plan.

Wherever possible use ORGANIC PRODUCE (including meat) to maximise the benefits of the detox effect: if this is not possible scrub the produce thoroughly.

Drinks – I recommend you drink a glass of liquid chlorophyll with or between every meal. Once diluted with water it has a minty refreshing taste. In addition to that drink water and diluted fruit juice or herbal or fruit teas. Hot water with lemon is great. Tea and coffee are excluded even if they are decaffeinated.

Snacks – fruits and vegetable nibbles as often as you want them. If you get hungry in-between meals or want a little bit more have some SynerProtein either plain as a shake or blended with some fruit. There are more snack ideas in the food and recipe section.

WHAT DO YOU NEED TO DO FIRST?

FIRST you need to sit down for 15 minutes or so and read through the whole programme – including recipes: next you need to make a shopping list for the items you will need. What you do eat is at least as important as what you don't eat on this plan, so shop well in advance so you are not caught out. If you want to use the herbal supplements to maximise weight loss and the beneficial health effects, see the "recommended products" page at the back of the book.

WHEN IS THE BEST TIME?

Next ask yourself when is a good time to do it – if you know the next 2 weeks are going to be manic at work or you have a houseful of guests or any stressful situation coming up – now is not the time. You need a moderate to quiet 2 weeks with no meals out, where you can really focus on you and getting yourself in shape. If you go astray – go back 2 days from where you were on the plan and resume from there.

BE DISCIPLINED

It will work it's tried and tested – I have done the hard part which is working out exactly what you need to eat: much as I would love to follow you around personally night and day for 2 weeks to constantly encourage and motivate you – I cant. You need to do that for yourself or with a friend. Doing the plan with others can be a great way to stay motivated.

ENERGY BOOSTING

There are enough energy giving foods in this plan for you to be able to sustain your normal activities – including exercise, so maintain your normal programme: however part of the reason for doing this is to get you to think about your body and how you should look after it – so if possible treat yourself to a massage or a steam or sauna. If that's not an option visit your local health shop and invest in some aromatherapy oils for the bath and have regular long soaks.

MOTIVATIONAL TIPS

A useful tip to remind yourself you are on a plan for a set period of time is this: find a nice piece of ribbon or string and tie it around your wrist the day you start the plan. Whenever someone offers you something that is not included on the plan or you are tempted to stray, look at the string and remind yourself that as long as you wear the string you WILL NOT stray from your target of achieving 2 weeks in complete control of everything you eat and drink. The ribbon is simply a reminder that you are working towards this goal, when you have completed the plan (and not before) you can remove the ribbon at the end of the 14th day. Also use the mind exercises described earlier in the book – see yourself as a healthy person saturating your body with healthy foods. Literally visualise all these vitamins and minerals pouring into your cells. Constantly tell yourself how healthy your diet is. Look at everything you eat over the next two weeks and make a mental note of what healthy food looks like.

DAY 1, 2 & 3

Breakfast
SynerProtein BLUE mixed in a blender with any soft fruit of your choice.

Or: bowl of porridge made with semi or skimmed milk and $\frac{1}{2}$ milk and water.
BLUE/PINK 1-teaspoon brown sugar or spoon (organic) honey, RED. Add a pinch of cinnamon or nutmeg for additional taste. Have with a large glass of fresh juice, (unsweetened) GREEN.

Alternatively have a bowl muesli. PINK. Home made if possible – see recipe, or a large smoothie, GREEN / BLUE. See recipes

If not having a smoothie have a large glass fruit juice – diluted with your chosen breakfast. GREEN

Lunch
Multigrain or wholemeal bread sandwich, PINK. Select BLUE filling from list, and add a generous handful of either watercress or raw spinach (or a mix of both) and fresh (organic) tomato, GREEN.

Dinner
Choose 1 BLUE food (see list) and serve with 3 portions of anything from the GREEN list i.e. any vegetables or 2/3rds plate serving of vegetable casserole, GREEN / PINK. (see recipes): for your PINK serving choose either new potatoes scrubbed and cooked or a jacket potato (organic if possible) scrubbed and cooked, or basmati or wholegrain rice.

Snacks
Unlimited fruit and vegetable nibbles GREEN or a glass of SynerProtein BLUE or a large dessert spoon of fresh nuts and or seeds, BLUE.

Fluid
Aim for at least 3 glasses of liquid chlorophyll and an additional 3–4 glasses of water per day, or diluted fresh fruit juice (unsweetened). Herbal teas or hot water and lemon also recommended.

Breakfast
SynerProtein BLUE, mixed in a blender with any soft fruit of your choice GREEN. Or: extra large bowl of fruit salad or at least 3 pieces/portions of fresh or tinned fruit (no added sugar) GREEN. 1 small/medium pot low fat bio-yoghurt BLUE, & a large glass of fresh unsweetened fruit juice – dilute to taste GREEN. Alternatively have a small smoothie GREEN / BLUE (see recipe) in place of yoghurt.

If not having a smoothie have a large glass of fruit juice – diluted with your chosen breakfast. GREEN

Lunch
Multigrain or wholemeal bread sandwich, PINK, select BLUE filling from list, and add a generous handful of either watercress or raw spinach (or a mix of both) and tomato, GREEN.

Dinner
Choose 1 BLUE food from the list and serve with 3 portions of GREEN (any vegetables) or 2/3rds plate serving of vegetable casserole GREEN / PINK (see recipes): and for your PINK serving choose either new potatoes scrubbed and cooked, or a jacket potato scrubbed and cooked, or basmati or wholegrain rice.

Snacks
Unlimited fruit and vegetable nibbles GREEN or a glass of SynerProtein BLUE/GREEN or a large dessert spoon of fresh nuts and or seeds, BLUE.

Fluid – Aim for at least 3 glasses of liquid chlorophyll and an additional 3-4 glasses of water per day, or diluted fresh fruit juice (unsweetened). Herbal teas or hot water and lemon also recommended.

Breakfast
SynerProtein BLUE mixed in a blender with any soft fruit of your choice GREEN. Or extra large bowl of fruit salad or at least 3 pieces/portions of fresh fruit GREEN & 1 small/medium pot low fat bio-yoghurt BLUE & a large glass fresh unsweetened fruit juice – dilute to taste, GREEN. Alternatively have a smoothie GREEN / BLUE (see recipes) in place of yoghurt.

If not having a smoothie have a large glass fruit juice – diluted with your chosen breakfast. GREEN

Lunch
Fresh homemade soup GREEN / BLUE (see recipes) in unlimited amounts

Dinner
Choose 1 BLUE food (see list) served with an extra large portion of fresh salad GREEN (see recipes) served with either new potatoes scrubbed and cooked or a jacket potato scrubbed and cooked or basmati or wholegrain rice PINK. For the salad dressing see recipe.

Snacks
Unlimited fruit and vegetable nibbles GREEN or a glass of SynerProtein BLUE/GREEN or a large dessert spoon of fresh nuts and or seeds, BLUE.

Fluid
Aim for at least 3 glasses of liquid chlorophyll and an additional 3-4 glasses of water per day, or diluted fresh fruit juice (unsweetened). Herbal teas or hot water and lemon also recommended.

Breakfast
SynerProtein BLUE mixed in a blender with any soft fruit of your choice GREEN. Or extra large bowl of fruit salad or at least 3 pieces/portions of fresh fruit GREEN & 1 small/medium pot low fat bio-yoghurt BLUE & a large glass fresh unsweetened fruit juice – dilute to taste, GREEN. Alternatively have a smoothie GREEN / BLUE (see recipes) in place of yoghurt.

If not having a smoothie have a large glass fruit juice – diluted with your chosen breakfast. GREEN

Lunch
Fresh homemade soup GREEN / BLUE (see recipes) in unlimited amounts

Dinner
Choose 1 BLUE food (see list) and serve with 3 portions of GREEN (any vegetables) or 2/3rds plate serving of vegetable casserole GREEN / PINK (see recipes): and for your PINK serving choose either new potatoes scrubbed and cooked or a jacket potato scrubbed and cooked or basmati or wholegrain rice.

- Vegetarians replace meat with 4-8 oz tofu or quorn.

Snacks
Unlimited fruit and vegetable nibbles GREEN or a glass of SynerProtein BLUE/GREEN or a large dessert spoon of fresh nuts and or seeds, BLUE.

Fluid
Aim for at least 3 glasses of liquid chlorophyll and an additional 3-4 glasses of water per day, or diluted fresh fruit juice (unsweetened). Herbal teas or hot water and lemon also recommended.

Breakfast

SynerProtein BLUE mixed in a blender with any soft fruit of your choice GREEN. Or extra large bowl of fruit salad or at least 3 pieces/portions of fresh fruit GREEN & 1 small/medium pot low fat bio-yoghurt BLUE & a large glass fresh unsweetened fruit juice – dilute to taste, GREEN. Alternatively have a smoothie GREEN / BLUE (see recipes) in place of yoghurt.

If not having a smoothie have a large glass fruit juice – diluted with your chosen breakfast. GREEN

Lunch

Multigrain or wholemeal bread sandwich PINK, select BLUE filling from list, and add a generous handful of either watercress or raw spinach (or a mix of both) and tomato, GREEN.

Dinner

Choose 1 BLUE food (see list) e.g. chicken breast, fish steak, or tofu and serve with 3 portions of GREEN (any vegetables) or 2/3rds plate serving of vegetable casserole GREEN / PINK (see recipes): and for your PINK serving choose either new potatoes scrubbed and cooked or a jacket potato scrubbed and cooked or basmati or wholegrain rice.

- Vegetarians replace meat with 4-8 oz tofu or quorn.

Snacks

Unlimited fruit and vegetable nibbles GREEN or a glass of SynerProtein BLUE/GREEN or a large dessert spoon of fresh nuts and or seeds, BLUE.

Fluid

Aim for at least 3 glasses of liquid chlorophyll and an additional 3-4 glasses of water per day, or diluted fresh fruit juice (unsweetened). Herbal teas or hot water and lemon also recommended.

RECIPES

All calorific values are approximate & may vary slightly according to size and ripeness of foods. Colour codes are shown to help you balance your intake.

Smoothies

For all smoothies simply put all the ingredients into a blender. For a refreshing drink add or serve over crushed ice.

GREEN
Sweet Berry Smoothie - 2 servings:

225g (8 oz) mixture of strawberries, raspberries & blueberries
2 kiwi fruit – peeled and chopped
150g carton low fat natural bio yoghurt
½ tablespoon clear organic honey

GREEN
Watermelon Smoothie – 2 servings

½ small watermelon (approx 1.5kg – 3 lb peeled and cubed)
150g carton low fat natural bio yoghurt.
Put all ingredients into a blender

GREEN
Strawberry Smoothie – 2 servings

450g ripe strawberries
Grated zest & juice of an orange
150g pot low fat bio yoghurt

GREEN
Mango & Banana Smoothie – 2 servings

½ large ripe mango – discard stone & chop
1 small banana chopped
150ml semi- skimmed milk
120ml fresh orange juice
2 tablespoons low fat frozen yoghurt

PINK
Homemade Energy Boost Muesli – 2 Servings
Add ⅓ pt semi skimmed milk @ 90 cal or a small/medium pot
very low fat bio yoghurt

Bran flakes 1 cup
Oat flakes 1 cup
Almonds 10-12
Chopped dates x 4
Raisins ½ cup
Sunflower seeds 2 tbsp
Sliced banana small

Choose all or some of the ingredients and mix together in a bowl. Allow approximately 60g of the combined ingredients for 1 serving, excluding fresh banana. Serve with 1/3 pint of skimmed or semi skimmed milk *or* a pot of low fat bio yoghurt.

Change or adapt the ingredients in all smoothies according to tastes and adjust calories accordingly

GREEN
Fresh Fruit Salad – 2 Servings

Honeydew melon ½
Strawberries 1 cup
Pineapple 1 cup
Grapes 1 cup
Kiwi x 1
Pear x 1

*You can use tinned pineapple in unsweetened juice, and use the juice to pour over all the fruit: Alternatively use some fresh unsweetened orange juice. If you like more flavour, add a pinch of nutmeg or cinnamon.

This combination can be made in advance and kept in the fridge for 2–3 days so make up a large bowl. If you are using apples or bananas you will need to add them daily. Experiment with different combinations depending on what's in season: any variety or combination of fruits will be fine.

Soups

Wherever possible use organic veg and be very tight on the amount of salt you use. The smallest pinch is sufficient & if you are using stock cube or bouillon then do not any add extra salt.

GREEN
Green Soup – 4 Servings

4 medium potatoes chopped
1 medium leek sliced
3 cups broccoli chopped
1-2 cloves garlic (depending on taste preference)
s&p
Sage for seasoning – $\frac{1}{2}$ tsp or to taste
Water
Veg or chicken stock cube or bouillon.

Boil leek and potatoes for about 15 mins and add the stock cube or bouillon. Add the broccoli sage and garlic and simmer for a further 15 mins. Add extra water if required to get required amount and thickness.

Can be served chunky or put through a processor for a smoother texture. Add extra water as required if end result is too thick.

GREEN
Mixed Vegetable Soup – 4 Servings

3 large carrots chopped
1 large parsnip chopped
2 cup turnip chopped
1 onion finely chopped
2-cup cabbage chopped
s&p
Coriander
Splash limejuice
Veg or chicken stock cube or bouillon.

Place all the veg into a large pan of boiling water add stock cube or bouillon: after 15 mins add s&p and coriander and simmer till soft, approx 20-25 mins in total. 5 mins before end add limejuice.

Can be served chunky or put through a processor for a smoother texture. Add extra water as required if end result is too thick.

GREEN
Carrot Courgette & Sweetcorn Soup – 4 Servings

2 large carrots chopped
2 courgettes chopped
1-cup sweet corn frozen
1 onion finely chopped
s&p
½-1tsp oregano
(Veg or chicken stock cube or bouillon if needed for extra flavour)

Place carrots into large pan of boiling water, cover and simmer for 10 mins. Add courgettes and onions and simmer a further 10 mins. Add sweetcorn s&p and oregano and simmer for 5 further mins.

Can be served chunky or put through a processor for a smoother texture. Add extra water as required if end result is too thick.

GREEN
Vegetable & Lentil Soup – 4 Servings

2 large carrots chopped
1 onion chopped
100g red lentils cooked as per packet instructions
2 sticks celery finely chopped
$\frac{1}{2}$ tsp cumin
$\frac{1}{2}$ tsp coriander
s&p
(Veg or chicken stock cube or bouillon if needed for extra flavour)

Add carrots (& celeriac if not using celery) to boiling water and simmer for 10 mins. Add onions (and celery if appropriate) and simmer for a further 5 mins. Add the lentils s&p and herbs and simmer a further 5 mins.

Can be served chunky or put through a processor for a smoother texture. Add extra water as required if end result is too thick.

Salads

Serve with anything from BLUE list

For all salads you may add some olives, or $\frac{1}{2}$ an avocado as these are excellent sources of Essential Fatty Acids (EFA's)

GREEN
Green Salad – 2 Servings

Iceberg lettuce – handful of leaves
1 Sliced courgette
100g Mange tout
100g Green beans
100g Watercress
1 cup Grapefruit segments (if tinned *not* in syrup)
$\frac{1}{2}$ Avocado

GREEN
Carrot & Orange Salad – 2 Servings

2 Carrots –grated
2 small oranges or mandarin segments (if tinned *not* in syrup)
2 cup Spinach leaves
1 Yellow pepper – sliced
1 stick Celery – finely chopped

GREEN
Chinese Salad – 2 Servings

1 cup Pineapple segments (if tinned *not* in syrup)
Iceberg lettuce handful of leaves
Chinese Leaf handful of leaves
2 Spring onions
1 cup Bean sprouts
4 inches Cucumber – cut into thin strips
1 tbsp of sesame seeds

GREEN
Red Salad – 2 Servings

2 cups Red cabbage finely chopped
2 Red apples (organic) chopped (with peel left on)
1 Chopped red onion
2 sticks Celery finely chopped
50g black olives

GREEN
Vegetable Salad – 2 Servings

2 cups Spinach leaves
1 cups Chopped broccoli
1 cups Chopped cauliflower
100g Mange tout
1 Sliced green or red peppers
4 large tomatoes 1 cup frozen peas (leave to defrost naturally in salad – do not cook).

NOTE – These are suggestions of items that go well together – you can either use them as they are or according to your preference mix and match the recipes adding in extra or leaving out where necessary. You can also vary the amounts you use for the salad dressing & vary the herbs you use according to your taste:

GREEN
Humus – makes 3 servings

400g tin chick peas drained & rinsed
150g low fat plain yoghurt
pinch black pepper
1 glove garlic crushed/chopped
lemon or lime juice to taste (a generous squeeze)
2 teaspoons (10 ml) sesame oil

Put all ingredients into a bowl and mash vigorously with a fork. Alternatively put in a blender for a smoother finish.

BLUE
Salad Dressing – makes 10 servings

2 fl oz Extra virgin olive oil
1-2 fl oz balsamic vinegar
1-2 fl oz orange juice
splash lemon/lime juice to taste
black pepper & either 1/2 tsp mustard powder or herb or spice of your choice e.g. mint, chopped coriander, parsley or garlic etc.

GREEN
Vegetable Casserole – makes 4 large servings

200g Potatoes
3 med/large Carrots
1 red onion
200g leeks
200g swede
200g parsnips
Tin chopped tomatoes
1 red pepper cut into 6 large pieces

1 yellow pepper cut into 6 large pieces
1 tin chick peas drained
50g marmite

Chop and place all the ingredients in an ovenproof dish, Cover with stock (use bouillon or stock cube) & stir in marmite. Put lid on or cover with foil & place in a medium high oven (approx 180-190) for 50-60 mins.

This recipe is ideal if you have a busy lifestyle as you can make a large pot – sufficient for a few days & microwave a portion as you need it.

BLUE
Sandwich Fillings and Portion Sizes
- Ham - 1-2 lean slices
- Chicken 1-2 lean slices
- Beef 1-2lean slices
- Turkey 1-2 lean slices
- Edam cheese 2-3 oz grated
- Brie 2-3oz
- Feta cheese 2-3oz
- 1 boiled egg
- Tinned tuna in spring water 65g (1/2 small 130g tin)
- Tinned pink salmon 100g (1/2 small 213g tin)
- 1 serving Home made humus (see recipe)
- $^{1}/_{2}$ cup raw spinach or watercress approx

BLUE FOODS
Portion size guidelines for meat: women 4-6oz /100 –170g, men 6-8 oz/170-230g

- Fillet steak griddled
- chicken breast roasted griddled or grilled
- turkey – light meat, roasted griddled or grilled
- wild red salmon griddled or grilled
- trout griddled or grilled
- swordfish steak griddled or grilled
- 4-6oz/100-170g tofu (soya bean) steamed
- 4-6oz /100-170g quorn

- 8-10 Almonds
- 6-8 whole Brazil nuts
- 1 cup cottage cheese
- 3-4oz /85-113g edam cheese
- 3-4 oz 85-113g Brie
- 3-4 oz 85-113g Feta cheese
- 2 boiled eggs
- 1 serving Home made humus

You should eat enough food so as NOT to be hungry. If you are hungry – have an extra glass of SynerProtein, a bowl of soup or some fruit or nuts and seeds. The emphasis is on if you are hungry – not if you are bored! ONLY eat when you are hungry and ONLY eat as much as you need to feel satisfied, NOT as much as it takes to "fill you up". Listen carefully to your body.

WHAT HAPPENS NEXT?

That is entirely up to you. Who do you want to be? What exactly will you achieve? I have emphasised all along that this is a book you DO not just a book you read. What have you already done, what else can you do? It's your choice.

I leave you with this story which was sent to me by a friend, I wish I could credit who wrote it, or even if it's true, I have no idea where it came from but it's a great story:

Michael's story

Michael was one of those guys you love to hate. He was always in such a good mood and always had something positive to say. If someone asked him how he was doing he would reply, "Hey if I were any better, I'd be twins". He was a natural motivator. If a colleague was having a bad day Michael was there giving them the positive side of the situation.

Seeing this style made me curious so one day I went to him and said "I don't get it, you can't be a positive person all the time. How do you do it?"

Michael replied, "Each morning I wake up and say to myself you have two choices today you can choose to be in a good mood or you can choose to be in a bad mood".

I choose to be in a good mood.

Each time something bad happens I can choose to be a victim or I can choose to learn from it.

I choose to learn from it.

Every time someone comes to me complaining I can accept their complaining or I can point out the positive side of life.

I choose the positive side of life.

"Yeah right" I protested "its not that easy".

"Yes it is" Michael said "life's all about choices" When you cut away all the junk every situation is a choice. All you do is choose how to react to any given situation.

You choose how people affect your mood, you choose to be in a good mood or a bad mood you choose to help others or not help others.

The bottom line is: its your choice how you live life.

I went away and reflected on what Michael had said. Soon after I moved to another division and away from where Michael worked, we lost touch but I often thought about what he said when making a choice about life rather than reacting to it.

Several years later I heard that Michael had been involved in a serious accident falling some sixty feet whilst climbing.

After 20 hours of surgery and a couple of months in Intensive care Michael was released from Hospital with rods in his back. I saw Michael some six months after the accident and asked how he was. He smiled (I knew what was coming) and replied, "If I were any better I'd be twins, want to see my scars?"

I said No but did ask him what went through his mind as the accident took place.

He responded " the first thing that went through my mind was the well being of my children, then as I lay on the ground I reminded myself I had a choice, I could choose to live or to die.

I chose to live.

"Weren't you scared?" I asked. Michael continued. "The Paramedics were great they kept telling me I would be fine but when they wheeled me into the A&E department I saw the expressions on the faces of the Doctors and Nurses then I got really scared".

"I saw in their eyes, *he's a dead man,* and I knew I needed to do something".

"So what did you do?" I enquired. "Well" he responded, "There was this big nurse who kept asking me questions and if I was allergic to anything". So I replied, "Yes"

The Doctors and Nurses stopped working waiting for my answer so I drew a breath and shouted "Gravity!!!!"

Over their laughter I told them "I am choosing to live, operate on me as though I am alive and not dead".

Michael lived, thanks to the skill of the Doctors, but also because of his amazing attitude.

I learned from Michael that every day we have a choice to live happily and fully and what's great is it's in our control it's our choice. We choose our attitude.

Attitude after all, is everything.

So don't worry about tomorrow, today should be full enough for you, and anyway isn't today the tomorrow you worried about yesterday

Recommended Products and Contact Details

Visit **www.powertochange.me.uk** for one to one appointments or treatments, or for link to Natures Sunshine to order recommended Products:

- Healthy Starter Pack (for detox)
- SynerProtein (for detox and daily use)
- Liquid Chlorophyll (for detox and daily use)
- Zambrosa (for detox and daily use)

Email: Sean Quigley TFT VT: *sean@tft-vt.com* for information on **TFT Voice Technology and Toxin Testing**.

www.diagnosemefirst.com for information on PCOS and Insulin resistance

www.ionizers.org for information on acid/alkaline balance and water purifiers.

www.kettlerdirect.co.uk for information on rebounders and other home exercise equipment.

For the WLIM Weekend 'Bootcamp', two-day TFT courses, self-hypnosis days, and other training and seminars, email info@powertochange.me.uk.

For more information, visit **www.powertochange.me.uk**

DAILY CHECK LIST   date_____

GREEN (MIN 6) FRUIT   [ ]   [ ]   [ ]

               VEG   [ ]   [ ]   [ ]   [ ]   [ ]   [ ]

PINK   (UP TO 4) BREAD/PASTA   [ ]   [ ]   [ ]

           RICE/CEREAL/POTATO

BLUE   (UP TO 5) MEAT/DAIRY/OILS   [ ]   [ ]   [ ]   [ ]   [ ]

                  NUTS/SEEDS

RED   MAX 250 CALS   [ ]   **EXERCISE TODAY**   **YES / NO**

DAILY CHECK LIST   date_____

GREEN (MIN 6) FRUIT   [ ]   [ ]   [ ]

               VEG   [ ]   [ ]   [ ]   [ ]   [ ]   [ ]

PINK   (UP TO 4) BREAD/PASTA   [ ]   [ ]   [ ]

           RICE/CEREAL/POTATO

BLUE   (UP TO 5) MEAT/DAIRY/OILS   [ ]   [ ]   [ ]   [ ]   [ ]

                  NUTS/SEEDS

RED   MAX 250 CALS   [ ]   **EXERCISE TODAY**   **YES / NO**

If you have the complete WLIM system a printable version is available on the 'Resource CD'.

The complete WEIGHT LOSS IN MIND system includes the WLIM book, and three audio CDs, specifically designed to enable YOU to change your mind, along with a resource CD containing 28 days worth of recipes to get you started and a 28 day workout programme. If you have only purchased the book, but would like the whole package, it is available from www.powertochange.me.uk.

Audio CDs

"Trance" is a way of allowing your unconscious mind to consider and make changes. It is a very individual experience: some people remember everything that was said during the trance consciously, others remember to forget what they don't need to remember consciously, safe in the knowledge that your unconscious knows.

These CDs have been designed to bring about the changes you already *want* to make; they are generic in many ways, as your unconscious already knows exactly what to do with the information in a way that's right for YOU. You will hear my voice primarily but also Sean's voice; this technique of double induction is very powerful.

Trance is a different experience for everyone, some people feel they have dozed off, others feel wide awake and very alert. YOU will be in control of what you are thinking and learning the whole time and your unconscious mind will ONLY change what is right for you to change.

For best results, read the first chapter of the book, at least up to page 20, and then begin to use the "Making Changes" audio CD. There is no limit to the number of times you will benefit from listening and following this audio guided trance. When you have read and completed the exercises in the book up to page 69, begin to listen to and follow the guided trance on the "Treasure Chest" CD. You will achieve maximum benefit from this audio guided trance, if you listen to it, and follow it, several times. There is no limit to the amount of times you can listen to and benefit from either of the aforementioned CDs, and you may find each time you listen, your unconscious makes more and more changes that will help you to lose weight in a way that's right for you. These changes will be further enhanced as you work through the exercises in the book.

"Relax and Change" can be used when you have installed some new behaviours or have new ways of thinking. As soon as you actively (either consciously or unconsciously) notice changes you have already started to make, or have read up to page 85, begin to play this CD regularly to reinforce those changes.

CD 1 Making Changes – designed to delete old behaviours and install new more beneficial ones. Find a time and place when you have time (approx 30 mins) to just sit or lie down and relax – undisturbed. This CD can be played repeatedly as many times as required, or in the future of you ever want a "top up".

CD 2 Treasure Chest – designed to help you LET GO of baggage, perhaps experiences, feelings or limiting beliefs, and replace them with new compelling skills and feelings. Find a time and place when you have time (approx 40 mins) to just sit or lie down and relax – undisturbed. This CD can be played repeatedly as many times as required, or in the future of you ever want a "top up".

CD 3 Relax and Change – designed to support and enhance anything, you have changed. It is designed (though not compulsory) to be listened to when you go to bed, there is no counting out of the trance and you may find it aids peaceful restful sleep.